MEMORY LOSS RECUPERATION COOKBOOK FOR SENIORS

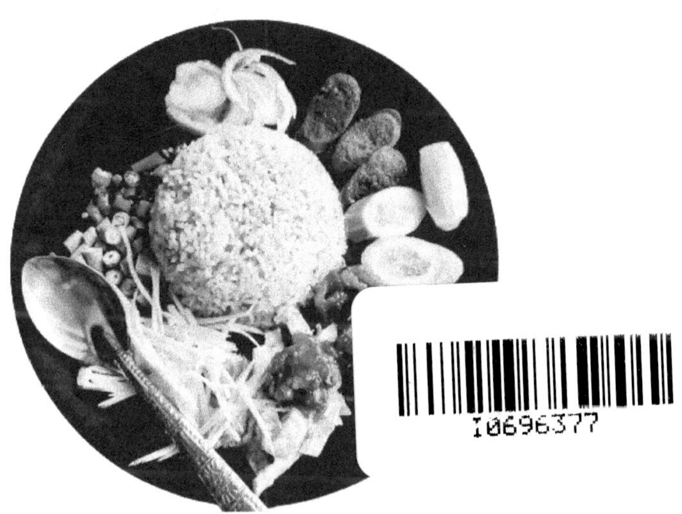

Unlock Cognitive Vitality with Proven Recipes for Alzheimer's Treatment and Prevention with Nutrient-Rich Dietary Suggestions

Anita Mark

DISCLAIMER

Acknowledgment

To those instrumental in bringing "The Memory Loss Recuperation Cookbook for Seniors" to life, sincere gratitude:

Seniors: Your resilience and wisdom have profoundly influenced this work, transforming it into a tribute to a lifetime of cherished memories.

Caregivers: The backbone of this project, your dedication and sacrifices are acknowledged with deep appreciation for the tireless efforts you contribute.

Families and Friends: As silent companions on this literary journey, your presence has enriched each shared memory, creating a book that resonates with shared experiences.

Healthcare Professionals: Grateful for your invaluable insights and commitment to the well-being of seniors; your expertise has shaped the essence of this book.

Culinary Explorers: Celebrating your passion in the kitchen, this book is a testament to the joy you bring, infusing every page with the spirit of culinary exploration.

Dedication

This Book is Dedicated to SENIORS with COGNITIVE CHALLENGES

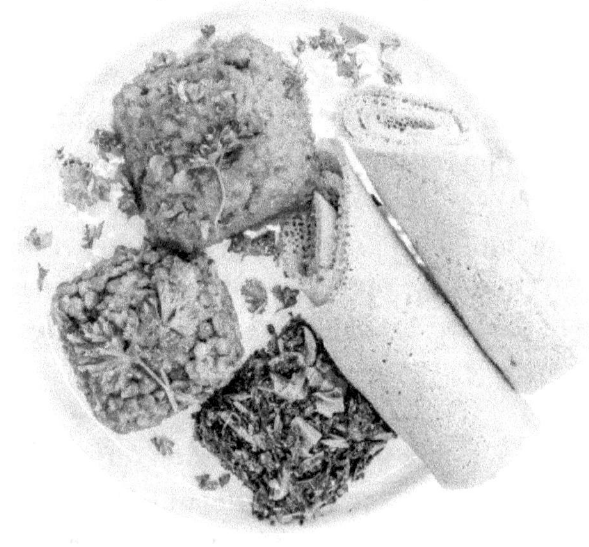

Table of Contents

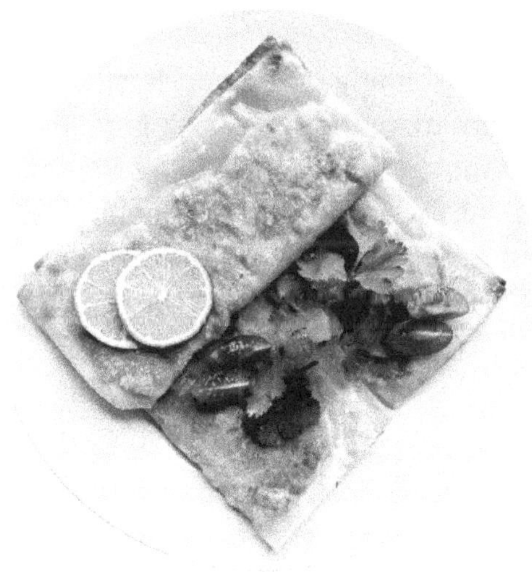

Introduction

In a world where memories could sometimes slip through the fingers like grains of sand, there exists a cookbook that has become a beacon of hope for countless seniors. It's not just a cookbook; it's a culinary journey that weaves together the intricate tapestry of flavors, nutrition, and memories. This is a story of how our "Memory Loss Recuperation Cookbook for Seniors for Seniors" has transformed the lives of readers, filling their hearts and minds with the warmth of delicious meals and the brilliance of cherished recollections.

Imagine an elderly couple, Mary and John, whose once-vibrant memories began to fade like the colors of a vintage photograph. Their life's journey had been remarkable, filled with shared laughter, adventures, and love. But as time passed, memory loss cast a shadow over their cherished moments.

Then, one day, their daughter Grace, an avid reader and caregiver, discovered the treasure trove that is our cookbook. Its pages held more than just recipes; they contained the promise of renewed connections and vibrant moments.

As Mary and John began to explore the recipes and wisdom within, something magical happened. The aroma of sizzling garlic, the sound of simmering soups, and the taste of carefully crafted dishes rekindled their passion for cooking together. It was as if each recipe had its own story, whispered by generations of caregivers, and now, shared by Mary and John.

With the help of the cookbook, Mary and John embarked on a culinary adventure, finding comfort in creating meals that nourished not only their bodies but also their memories. They noticed a spark in each other's eyes as they reminisced about the ingredients and steps to prepare a meal. Through this shared journey, they forged new memories that intertwined with their past, creating a richer tapestry of their life story.

The power of this cookbook was not confined to Mary and John. As they hosted family dinners and shared their newfound knowledge with friends, they witnessed the impact it had on others battling memory loss. Their gatherings became an oasis of connection, filled with laughter and conversations.

The "Memory Loss Recuperation Cookbook for Seniors for Seniors" is more than just a collection of recipes; it is a guide to reignite the flames of memory, a companion for seniors and their loved ones in the journey of rediscovery.

In the pages of this book, you'll find not only the ingredients for delicious meals but also the ingredients for rekindling the warmth of shared stories and cherished moments. Join us in this culinary adventure that has enlightened, encouraged, and educated seniors, showing them that memory loss is not the end but the beginning of a new chapter filled with flavor, love, and joy.

Understanding Memory in Seniors

Understanding memory loss in seniors is crucial for providing appropriate care and support to aging individuals. Memory loss is a common concern among the elderly, and it can be caused by various factors, including normal aging, underlying health conditions, or neurodegenerative diseases like Alzheimer's. Here's a comprehensive overview:

1. Normal Age-Related Memory Changes:
   - It's essential to recognize that some degree of memory decline is a natural part of aging. Older adults may experience occasional forgetfulness, such as misplacing keys or having difficulty recalling names, but these memory lapses do not significantly impact daily life.

2. Mild Cognitive Impairment (MCI):
   - MCI is a condition that lies between normal age-related memory changes and more severe cognitive decline. It involves noticeable memory problems but does not interfere significantly with daily activities.

3. Alzheimer's Disease:

The most typical cause of dementia in older adults is Alzheimer's disease. It is characterized by the progressive loss of memory, cognitive function, and the ability to perform everyday tasks. Early diagnosis and intervention are crucial.

4. Other Types of Dementia:

- Dementia can result from various underlying conditions, including vascular dementia, Lewy body dementia, and frontotemporal dementia. Each type has distinct symptoms and characteristics.

5. Factors Contributing to Memory Loss:

- Various factors can contribute to memory loss, including chronic health conditions, medication side effects, depression, anxiety, and sleep disorders. It is imperative to recognise and deal with these root causes.

6. Preventive Measures:

- Seniors can take proactive steps to maintain cognitive health. This includes staying mentally and socially active, engaging in regular physical activity, maintaining a balanced diet, and managing chronic health conditions.

7. Diagnosis and Evaluation:

- If memory loss is a concern, it's crucial to seek a professional evaluation. A healthcare provider can assess memory function, perform cognitive tests, and order imaging or laboratory tests if needed.

8. Treatment and Care:

Depending on the major causes, memory loss has different treatments.For Alzheimer's and some forms of dementia, there is no cure, but interventions can help manage symptoms and enhance quality of life.

9. Support for Caregivers:

- Caregivers play a vital role in providing emotional and practical support to seniors with memory loss. Caregiver well-being and support are essential to ensure the best care for their loved ones.

10. Community Resources:

- There are various community resources, such as memory care programs, senior centers, and support groups, designed to provide assistance and social engagement for seniors with memory loss.

Understanding memory loss in seniors involves recognizing its various forms, causes, and the importance of early detection and intervention. With appropriate care, support, and proactive measures, seniors can continue to lead fulfilling lives and maintain cognitive well-being.

The Importance of Nutrition for Brain Health

Nutrition plays a pivotal role in brain health, and it's especially critical for seniors. The brain is an organ that requires a constant supply of nutrients to function optimally. Here's why nutrition is essential for brain health, particularly in aging individuals:

1. Cognitive Function: Proper nutrition is vital for maintaining cognitive function. Nutrients like omega-3 fatty acids, antioxidants, and B vitamins support memory, reasoning, and problem-solving abilities.

2. Neuroplasticity: The brain's ability to adapt and form new connections, known as neuroplasticity, relies on adequate nutrition. Nutrients like choline, found in eggs and lean meats, are essential for this process.

3. Energy Supply: The brain is an energy-intensive organ, and it relies on a steady supply of glucose from carbohydrates. For the brain to function at its best, blood sugar levels must remain stable.

4. Inflammation Reduction: A diet rich in anti-inflammatory foods, such as fruits, vegetables, and omega-3-rich fish, can reduce inflammation in the brain, which is linked to cognitive decline.

5. Antioxidants: Antioxidants, found in foods like berries and dark leafy greens, help protect brain cells from oxidative stress and damage.

6. Heart-Brain Connection: A heart-healthy diet, low in saturated fats and high in fruits, vegetables, and whole grains, supports healthy blood vessels, which, in turn, promote good blood flow to the brain.

7. Mood and Emotional Well-Being: Nutritional deficiencies can contribute to mood disorders and depression, which can impact cognitive health. Nutrients like vitamin D and omega-3s play a role in mood regulation.

8. Protection Against Neurodegenerative Diseases: Certain nutrients, such as curcumin in turmeric, may have protective effects against neurodegenerative diseases like Alzheimer's.

9. Gut-Brain Connection: Emerging research highlights the connection between gut health and brain health. A diet rich in fiber and probiotics can support a healthy gut microbiome, which may benefit cognitive function.

10. Hydration: Proper hydration is essential for brain function. Dehydration can lead to cognitive impairments, so seniors should ensure they drink enough water.

11. Weight Management: Maintaining a healthy weight through balanced nutrition supports overall health, including brain health. Cognitive decline is associated with obesity.

12. Nutritional Needs in Seniors: Seniors may have different nutritional needs due to changes in metabolism and appetite. Ensuring they receive adequate nutrients, including calcium and vitamin D for bone health, is essential.

13. Anti-Aging Effects: Some nutrients and dietary patterns, such as the Mediterranean diet rich in olive oil, can have anti-aging effects and may reduce the risk of age-related cognitive decline.

14. Dietary Considerations for Memory Loss: Seniors with memory loss or dementia may benefit from diets like the MIND diet, which emphasizes brain-boosting foods like leafy greens and berries.

15. Preventing Malnutrition: Seniors are at risk of malnutrition, which can have a significant impact on cognitive health. Adequate nutrition is vital to prevent malnutrition.

A balanced and nutritious diet, rich in a variety of foods, can have a profound impact on brain health. Seniors are encouraged to consult with healthcare providers or dietitians to tailor their nutrition to their specific needs and promote cognitive vitality as they age.

Chapter 1: Breakfast Recipes

Blueberry Oatmeal Breakfast Bowl

Time of Preparation: 15 minutes

Ingredients:
- 1/2 cup old-fashioned rolled oats
- One cup of unsweetened almond milk (or any other desired milk)
- 1/2 cup fresh blueberries
- 1 tablespoon maple syrup or honey (extra sweetening optional)
- 1 tablespoon chia seeds
- 1/4 teaspoon vanilla extract
- 1 tablespoon chopped nuts (e.g., almonds or walnuts)
- 1 teaspoon ground flaxseeds
- A pinch of cinnamon (optional)

Method of Preparation:
1. In a saucepan, combine the rolled oats and almond milk.
2. Bring the mixture to a gentle boil, then reduce heat to a simmer.
3. Stir occasionally and cook for about 5-7 minutes until the oats are creamy and cooked to your desired consistency.
4. Remove from heat and stir in the vanilla extract and chia seeds.

5. Let the oatmeal sit for a couple of minutes to thicken.

6. Transfer the oatmeal to a bowl and top with fresh blueberries, honey or maple syrup (if desired), chopped nuts, ground flaxseeds, and a pinch of cinnamon.

Nutritional Benefits for Seniors:

- Oats: Rich in fiber and complex carbohydrates, oats provide sustained energy and help stabilize blood sugar levels.

- Almond Milk: A source of healthy fats and vitamin E, which are beneficial for brain health.

- Blueberries: Packed with antioxidants that protect brain cells from oxidative damage and may improve cognitive function.

- Chia Seeds: High in omega-3 fatty acids, fiber, and protein, chia seeds support brain function and promote a feeling of fullness.

- Nuts (Almonds or Walnuts): Contain healthy fats, vitamin E, and antioxidants, which are linked to cognitive benefits.

- Flaxseeds: Provide omega-3 fatty acids, fiber, and lignans, which support brain and heart health.

- Cinnamon: May help improve cognitive function and provide a dash of flavor.

- Honey or Maple Syrup (Optional): Natural sweeteners that add a touch of sweetness without spiking blood sugar levels.

This Blueberry Oatmeal Breakfast Bowl is not only a delightful morning treat but also a nutritious choice for seniors. It offers a mix of brain-boosting ingredients, including antioxidants, omega-3 fatty acids, and fiber, all of which contribute to cognitive well-being.

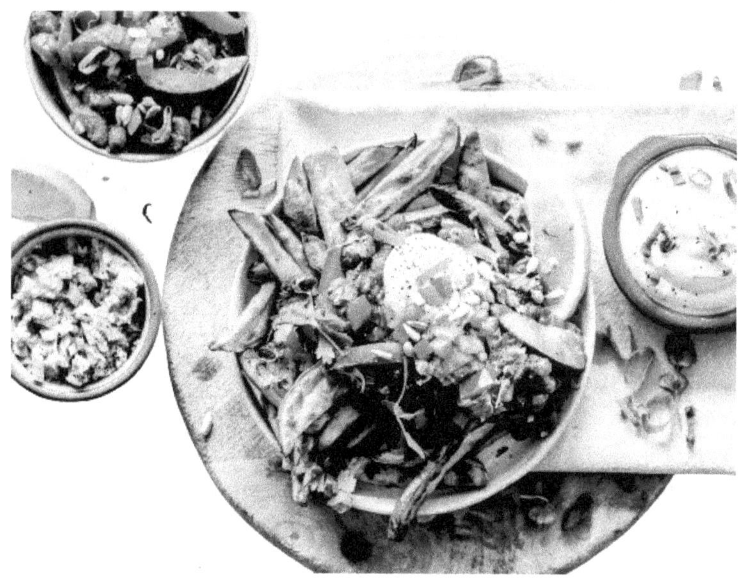

Spinach and Feta Omelette

Time of Preparation: 10 minutes

Ingredients:
- 2 large eggs
- 1/4 cup fresh spinach, chopped
- 2 tablespoons crumbled feta cheese
- 1 tablespoon olive oil
- Salt and pepper to taste
- Optional garnish of fresh herbs, such as parsley or basil

Method of Preparation:
1. Whisk the eggs until thoroughly combined in a bowl, Put some salt and pepper on it for seasoning.
2. In medium-sized nonstick skillet, heat olive oil.
3. Add the chopped spinach to the skillet and sauté for 1-2 minutes until wilted.
4. Pour the beaten eggs into the skillet, ensuring an even distribution.
5. Let the eggs cook for a minute, or until the edges begin to set, without stirring.
6. Sprinkle the crumbled feta cheese evenly over one half of the omelette.
7. Gently fold the other half of the omelette over the cheese, creating a half-moon shape.
8. Continue cooking for another minute or until the eggs are fully set and the cheese is slightly melted.

9. Slide the omelette onto a plate, garnish with fresh herbs if desired, and serve.

Nutritional Benefits for Seniors:
- Eggs: A source of choline and B vitamins that support brain function.
- Spinach: Rich in folate, vitamin K, and antioxidants, spinach supports cognitive health and may help reduce the risk of cognitive decline.
- Feta Cheese: Provides calcium and protein, which are essential for overall bone and muscle health in seniors.
- Olive Oil: Contains monounsaturated fats and antioxidants that promote heart and brain health.
- Fresh Herbs: Optional for flavor and added antioxidants.

This Spinach and Feta Omelette is a quick, tasty, and nutritious breakfast option for seniors. It offers a combination of protein, vitamins, and healthy fats that contribute to overall well-being, including cognitive health.

Whole Grain Pancakes with Berry Compote

Time of Preparation: 25 minutes

Ingredients:

For the Whole Grain Pancakes:
- 1 cup whole wheat flour
- 1/2 cup oat flour
- 2 tablespoons ground flaxseeds
- 2 teaspoons baking powder
- 1/2 teaspoon baking soda
- 1/4 teaspoon salt
- One cup of unsweetened almond milk (or any other desired milk)
- 1 large egg
- 1 tablespoon maple syrup or honey (extra sweetening optional)
- 1 teaspoon vanilla extract

For the Berry Compote:
- 1 cup mixed berries (e.g., blueberries, strawberries, raspberries)
- 1 tablespoon honey or maple syrup
- 1/2 teaspoon lemon juice

Method of Preparation:

For the Whole Grain Pancakes:
1. In a large bowl, combine the whole wheat flour, oat flour, ground flaxseeds, baking powder, baking soda, and salt.
2. In a separate bowl, whisk together the almond milk, egg, honey or maple syrup (if using), and vanilla extract.
3. Add the wet mixture to the dry mixture and stir just until blended. Leave some lumps; overmixing is not necessary.
4. Heat a non-stick skillet or griddle over medium heat and lightly grease it with cooking spray or a small amount of oil.
5. Pour 1/4 cup of pancake batter onto the skillet for each pancake.
6. Cook until bubbles form on the surface and the edges appear set, then flip and cook the other side until golden brown.
7. Repeat until all the batter is used, keeping the cooked pancakes warm.

For the Berry Compote:
1. In a small saucepan, combine the mixed berries, honey or maple syrup, and lemon juice.
2. Cook over low heat, stirring occasionally, until the berries break down and the mixture thickens, about 5-7 minutes.
3. Turn off the heat source and let it to cool down a little.

To Serve:
Place a stack of whole grain pancakes on a plate and top them with the warm berry compote.

Nutritional Benefits for Seniors:

Whole Grain Pancakes:
- Whole Wheat and Oat Flours: Rich in fiber, vitamins, and minerals that support heart and digestive health.
- Flaxseeds: Provide omega-3 fatty acids and additional fiber for brain and heart health.
- Almond Milk: Contains vitamin E and healthy fats beneficial for cognitive health.
- Honey or Maple Syrup (Optional): Natural sweeteners that add a touch of sweetness without spiking blood sugar levels.

Berry Compote:
- Mixed Berries: Packed with antioxidants and vitamins that protect brain cells and promote cognitive function.
- Honey or Maple Syrup: Optional natural sweeteners that enhance flavor.
This Whole Grain Pancakes with Berry Compote recipe is a delightful and nutritious breakfast option for seniors. It combines the goodness of whole grains and antioxidant-rich berries, offering a wholesome start to the day while supporting brain and overall health.

<u>Chia Seed Pudding with Almonds and Berries</u>

10 minutes of preparation time, plus chilling time

Ingredients:
- 1/4 cup chia seeds
- One cup of unsweetened almond milk (or any other desired milk)
- 1 tablespoon maple syrup or honey (extra sweetening optional)
- 1/4 teaspoon vanilla extract
- 1/4 cup sliced almonds
- 1/2 cup of mixed berries, such as raspberries, strawberries, and blueberries
- Fresh mint leaves for garnish (optional)

Method of Preparation:
1. In a bowl, combine the chia seeds, almond milk, honey or maple syrup (if using), and vanilla extract.
2. Stir the mixture thoroughly, making sure the chia seeds are well incorporated.
3. Cover the bowl and refrigerate for at least 3-4 hours, or overnight. By doing this, the liquid may be absorbed by the chia seeds, giving the mixture a pudding-like texture.
4. When ready to serve, give the chia pudding a good stir to ensure an even texture.
5. Divide the pudding into serving bowls or glasses.

6. Top each portion with sliced almonds and mixed berries.
7. If you'd like, garnish with freshly chopped mint leaves.

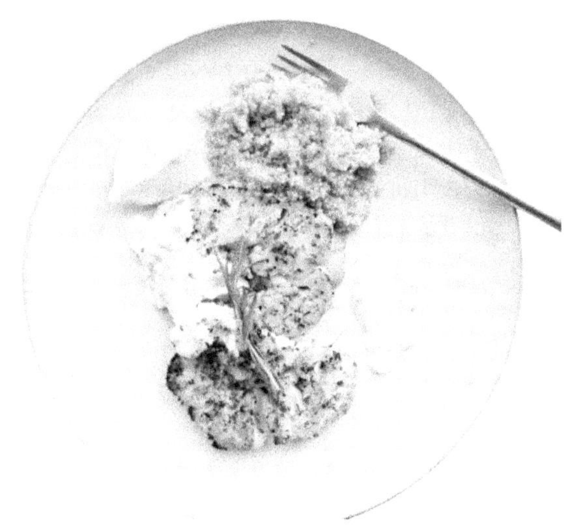

Nutritional Benefits for Seniors:
- Chia Seeds: High in fiber, omega-3 fatty acids, and protein, chia seeds promote brain health, satiety, and digestive well-being.
- Almond Milk: Provides vitamin E and healthy fats that support cognitive function and heart health.
- Honey or Maple Syrup (Optional): Natural sweeteners that add a touch of sweetness without causing spikes in blood sugar levels.

- Berries: Rich in antioxidants and vitamins that protect brain cells from oxidative damage and may improve cognitive function.
- Sliced Almonds: Contain healthy fats, protein, and vitamin E, which are linked to cognitive benefits.

This Chia Seed Pudding with Almonds and Berries is a simple and nutritious dessert or snack for seniors. It offers a delightful combination of brain-boosting chia seeds, almonds, and antioxidant-rich berries, making it a perfect treat that supports cognitive and overall health.

Avocado and Salmon Breakfast Toast

Time of Preparation: 15 minutes

Ingredients:
- 2 slices of whole-grain bread
- 1 ripe avocado
- 4 ounces smoked salmon
- 1 tablespoon lemon juice
- 1 tablespoon olive oil
- Salt and pepper to taste
- Fresh dill or chives for garnish (optional)

Method of Preparation:
1. Toast the whole-grain bread pieces until they reach the desired crispness.

2. Scoop the flesh from the ripe avocado into a dish, chop it in half, and remove the pit while the bread is toasting.

3. Mash the avocado with lemon juice, olive oil, salt, and pepper to create a smooth, creamy spread.

4. Once the toast is ready, spread the mashed avocado mixture evenly on each slice.

5. Layer the smoked salmon on top of the avocado spread.

6. Garnish with fresh dill or chives, if desired.

7. Serve immediately.

Nutritional Benefits for Seniors:

- Whole-Grain Bread: Provides complex carbohydrates and fiber for sustained energy and digestive health.

- Avocado: Rich in healthy monounsaturated fats, vitamin E, and antioxidants that support brain and heart health.

- Smoked Salmon: A source of omega-3 fatty acids and high-quality protein that are essential for cognitive and muscle health.

- Lemon Juice: Adds a burst of vitamin C, which is beneficial for overall health.

- Olive Oil: Contains monounsaturated fats and antioxidants that promote cognitive and heart health.

- Fresh Dill or Chives (Optional): Herbs that enhance flavor and provide additional antioxidants.

This Avocado and Salmon Breakfast Toast is a delectable and nutrient-rich way to start the day. It combines the brain-boosting benefits of omega-3 fatty acids from salmon and the healthy fats from avocado, all served on whole-grain toast for added fiber. It's a perfect breakfast choice for seniors.

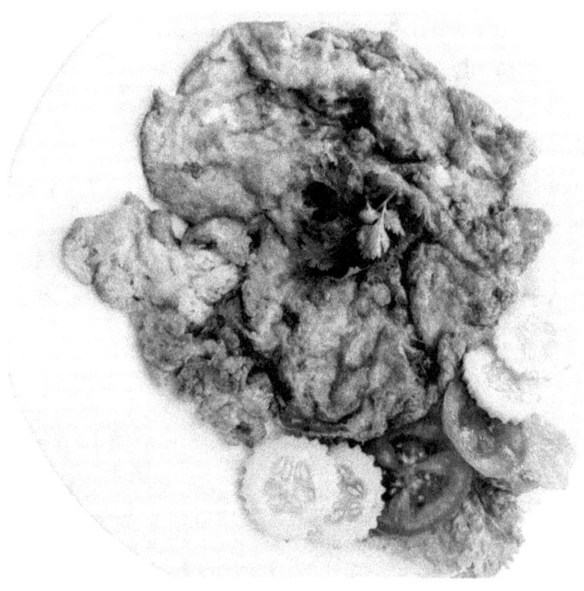

Chapter 2: Smoothies and Drinks

Nutty Banana Smoothie

Time of Preparation: 5 minutes

Ingredients:
- 1 ripe banana
- 1/4 cup plain Greek yogurt
- 1/4 cup unsweetened almond milk (or milk of choice)
- 2 tablespoons almond butter
- 1 tablespoon ground flaxseeds
- 1 teaspoon honey (optional for sweetness)
- 1/4 teaspoon cinnamon
- Ice cubes (optional)

Method of Preparation:
1. Peel the ripe banana and place it in a blender.
2. Add the plain Greek yogurt, unsweetened almond milk, almond butter, ground flaxseeds, honey (if using), and cinnamon.
3. If you prefer a colder smoothie, you can add a handful of ice cubes.
4. Process the mixture in a blender until it's creamy and smooth.
5. Taste and adjust the sweetness if necessary by adding more honey.

6. Pour the smoothie into a glass and serve immediately.

Nutritional Benefits for Seniors:
- Banana: A good source of potassium, vitamin B6, and dietary fiber that supports heart health and cognitive function.
- Greek Yogurt: Provides protein, probiotics, and calcium, which are essential for muscle, digestive, and bone health.
- Almond Milk: Contains vitamin E and healthy fats that support brain health.
- Almond Butter: High in healthy fats, protein, and vitamin E, which promote cognitive and heart health.
- Flaxseeds: Offer omega-3 fatty acids, fiber, and lignans, contributing to brain and heart health.
- Honey (Optional): A natural sweetener that adds sweetness without spiking blood sugar levels.
- Cinnamon: May help improve cognitive function and adds a dash of flavor.

This Nutty Banana Smoothie is a delicious and nutritious beverage for seniors. It incorporates the creaminess of banana, the goodness of Greek yogurt, and the brain-boosting properties of almond butter and flaxseeds. It's a quick and satisfying way to enjoy a wholesome snack or breakfast.

<u>Green Tea and Berry Smoothie</u>

Time of Preparation: 10 minutes

Ingredients:
-1 cup of cold-brewed green tea
- 1/2 cup of mixed berries, such as raspberries, strawberries, and blueberries
- 1/2 banana
- 1/2 cup plain Greek yogurt
- 1 tablespoon honey (optional for sweetness)
- Ice cubes (optional)
- Fresh mint leaves for garnish (optional)

Method of Preparation:
1. Brew a cup of green tea and let it cool to room temperature.
2. In a blender, combine the brewed and cooled green tea, mixed berries, half a banana, plain Greek yogurt, and honey (if using).
3. If you prefer a colder smoothie, you can add a handful of ice cubes.
4. Process all the ingredients in a blender until they are smooth and well mixed.
5. Taste and adjust the sweetness if necessary by adding more honey.
6. Pour the smoothie into a glass, garnish with fresh mint leaves (if desired), and serve.

Nutritional Benefits for Seniors:

- Green Tea: Contains antioxidants and L-theanine, which may support brain health and cognitive function.
- Mixed Berries: Packed with antioxidants and vitamins that protect brain cells from oxidative damage and may improve cognitive function.
- Banana: A good source of potassium, vitamin B6, and dietary fiber that supports heart health and cognitive function.
- Greek Yogurt: Provides protein, probiotics, and calcium, essential for muscle, digestive, and bone health.
- Honey (Optional): A natural sweetener that adds sweetness without spiking blood sugar levels.

This Green Tea and Berry Smoothie is a refreshing and nutritious beverage for seniors. It combines the brain-boosting properties of green tea with the antioxidant-rich nature of mixed berries, making it a delightful choice to support cognitive and overall health

Coconut and Kale Power Smoothie

Time of Preparation: 10 minutes

Ingredients:
- 1 cup unsweetened coconut milk (or milk of choice)
- 1 cup finely cut stem-free kale leaves
- 1/2 banana
- 1/4 cup shredded unsweetened coconut

- 1 tablespoon almond butter
- 1 tablespoon chia seeds
- 1 teaspoon honey (optional for sweetness)
- Ice cubes (optional)

Method of Preparation:
1. In a blender, combine the unsweetened coconut milk, chopped kale, half a banana, shredded unsweetened coconut, almond butter, chia seeds, and honey (if using).
2. If you prefer a colder smoothie, you can add a handful of ice cubes.
3. Process everything in a blender until it's smooth and well mixed.
4. Taste and adjust the sweetness if necessary by adding more honey.
5. Pour the smoothie into a glass and serve.

Nutritional Benefits for Seniors:
- Coconut Milk: Contains healthy fats and medium-chain triglycerides that support cognitive function and may help manage weight.
- Kale: A nutrient powerhouse, kale is rich in vitamins, minerals, and antioxidants that promote brain health and overall well-being.
- Banana: A good source of potassium, vitamin B6, and dietary fiber that supports heart health and cognitive function.
- Shredded Coconut: Provides healthy fats and fiber that can enhance brain and digestive health.

- Almond Butter: High in healthy fats, protein, and vitamin E, promoting cognitive and heart health.
- Chia Seeds: Offer omega-3 fatty acids, fiber, and protein, contributing to brain and digestive health.
- Honey (Optional): A natural sweetener that adds sweetness without spiking blood sugar levels.

This Coconut and Kale Power Smoothie is a vibrant and nutrient-packed beverage for seniors. It combines the creaminess of coconut milk with the powerhouse of nutrients from kale and chia seeds, making it a wonderful choice to support cognitive and overall health.

Spinach and Blueberry Superfood Smoothie

Time of Preparation: 10 minutes

Ingredients:
- 1 cup fresh spinach leaves
- 1/2 cup blueberries (fresh or frozen)
- 1/2 banana
- 1/2 cup plain Greek yogurt
- 1 tablespoon chia seeds
- 1 teaspoon honey (optional for sweetness)
- Ice cubes (optional)

Method of Preparation:

1. In a blender, combine the fresh spinach leaves, blueberries, half a banana, plain Greek yogurt, chia seeds, and honey (if using).
2. If you prefer a colder smoothie, you can add a handful of ice cubes.
3. Process everything in a blender until it's smooth and well mixed.
4. Taste and adjust the sweetness if necessary by adding more honey.
5. Pour the smoothie into a glass and serve.

Nutritional Benefits for Seniors:
- Spinach: Rich in folate, vitamin K, and antioxidants, spinach supports cognitive health and may help reduce the risk of cognitive decline.
- Blueberries: Packed with antioxidants that protect brain cells from oxidative damage and may improve cognitive function.
- Banana: A good source of potassium, vitamin B6, and dietary fiber that supports heart health and cognitive function.
- Greek Yogurt: Provides protein, probiotics, and calcium, essential for muscle, digestive, and bone health.
- Chia Seeds: Offer omega-3 fatty acids, fiber, and protein, contributing to brain and digestive health.
- Honey (Optional): A natural sweetener that adds sweetness without spiking blood sugar levels.

This Spinach and Bluecberry Superfood Smoothie is a vibrant and nutritious beverage for seniors. It combines the brain-boosting benefits of spinach and blueberries with the creaminess of Greek yogurt, making it a delightful choice to support cognitive and overall health.

Citrus and Ginger Brain Booster Juice

Time of Preparation: 10 minutes

Ingredients:
- 2 oranges, peeled and segmented
- 1 lemon, peeled and segmented
- 1 little, peeled piece of fresh ginger, about one inch in size
- 1 carrot, peeled and chopped
- 1/2 cup water
- 1 teaspoon honey (optional for sweetness)
- Ice cubes (optional)

Method of Preparation:
1. In a blender, combine the orange segments, lemon segments, fresh ginger, chopped carrot, and water.
2. If you prefer a colder juice, you can add a handful of ice cubes.
3. Blend all the ingredients until the juice is smooth.
4. Taste and adjust the sweetness if necessary by adding honey.
5. Pour the juice into a glass and serve immediately.

Nutritional Benefits for Seniors:

- Oranges: Rich in vitamin C and antioxidants, oranges support brain health and immune function.
- Lemon: Provides vitamin C and citrus bioflavonoids that protect brain cells and promote cognitive function.
- Ginger: Contains anti-inflammatory properties and may improve cognitive function.
- Carrot: High in beta-carotene, vitamins, and fiber, which are beneficial for brain and digestive health.
- Honey (Optional): A natural sweetener that adds sweetness without spiking blood sugar levels.

This Citrus and Ginger Brain Booster Juice is a zesty and nutritious beverage for seniors. It combines the cognitive benefits of citrus fruits and the potential brain-boosting properties of ginger. It's a refreshing choice to support cognitive and overall health.

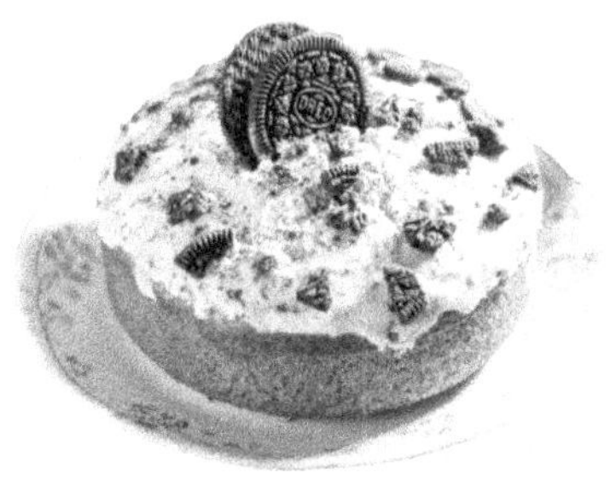

Chapter 3: Salads and Appetizers

Walnut and Mixed Greens Salad

Time of Preparation: 15 minutes

Ingredients:

For the Salad:
- Four cups of mixed greens, such as romaine, spinach and rocket
- 1/2 cup chopped walnuts
- 1/4 cup crumbled feta cheese
- 1/4 red onion, thinly sliced
- 1/2 cup cherry tomatoes, halved

For the Dressing:
- 2 tablespoons extra-virgin olive oil
- 1 tablespoon balsamic vinegar
- 1 teaspoon honey
- Salt and pepper to taste

Method of Preparation:
1. In a large salad bowl, combine the mixed greens, chopped walnuts, crumbled feta cheese, thinly sliced red onion, and cherry tomatoes.

2. In a separate small bowl, whisk together the extra-virgin olive oil, balsamic vinegar, honey, salt, and pepper to create the dressing.
3. Pour the dressing over the salad.
4. Toss the salad to ensure the ingredients are well coated with the dressing.
5. Serve immediately.

Nutritional Benefits for Seniors:
- Mixed Greens: Rich in vitamins, minerals, and antioxidants that support brain health and overall well-being.
- Walnuts: Provide healthy fats, antioxidants, and omega-3 fatty acids that may promote cognitive function and heart health.
- Feta Cheese: A source of calcium and protein, which are essential for bone and muscle health in seniors.
- Red Onion: Contains antioxidants and anti-inflammatory compounds that may support cognitive health.
- Cherry Tomatoes: Rich in vitamins, minerals, and antioxidants that protect brain cells and promote cognitive function.
- Olive Oil: Contains monounsaturated fats and antioxidants that support cognitive function and heart health.
- Honey: A natural sweetener that adds sweetness without spiking blood sugar levels.

This Walnut and Mixed Greens Salad is a delightful and nutritious choice for seniors. It combines the brain-boosting benefits of mixed greens and walnuts with the creamy texture of feta cheese. The flavorful dressing adds a touch of sweetness and tang, making it a wholesome addition to your meals.

Roasted Beet and Citrus Salad

Time of Preparation: 45 minutes

Ingredients:

For the Salad:
- 2-3 medium beets (red and/or golden)
- 2 oranges (e.g., navel or blood oranges)
- 1 grapefruit (pink or red grapefruit)
- 4 cups mixed greens (e.g., arugula, spinach, or baby greens)
- 1/4 cup crumbled goat cheese
- 1/4 cup chopped pecans or walnuts
- Fresh mint leaves for garnish (optional)

For the Dressing:
- 2 tablespoons extra-virgin olive oil
- 1 tablespoon balsamic vinegar
- 1 tablespoon honey
- Salt and pepper to taste

Method of Preparation:
1. Preheat your oven to 400°F (200°C).

2. Wash and peel the beets, then wrap them individually in aluminum foil. Place them on a baking sheet and roast for about 30-40 minutes or until they are tender when pierced with a fork. Allow them to cool.

3. While the beets are roasting, prepare the citrus fruits. Peel and segment the oranges and grapefruit, collecting any juice in a separate bowl.

4. Once the beets are cool, cut them into bite-sized pieces.

5. In a large salad bowl, combine the roasted beet pieces, citrus segments, mixed greens, crumbled goat cheese, and chopped pecans or walnuts.

6. In a separate small bowl, whisk together the extra-virgin olive oil, balsamic vinegar, honey, salt, and pepper to create the dressing.

7. Drizzle the dressing over the salad and toss to combine.

8. If you'd like, garnish with freshly chopped mint leaves.

9. Serve immediately.

Nutritional Benefits for Seniors:

- Beets: High in nitrates that may enhance blood flow to the brain and support cognitive function.

- Oranges and Grapefruit: Rich in vitamin C and antioxidants that protect brain cells from oxidative damage and promote cognitive function.

- Mixed Greens: Provide vitamins, minerals, and antioxidants that support brain health and overall well-being.

- Goat Cheese: A source of calcium and protein, which are essential for bone and muscle health in seniors.

- Pecans or Walnuts: Contain healthy fats, antioxidants, and omega-3 fatty acids that may promote cognitive function and heart health.
- Olive Oil: Contains monounsaturated fats and antioxidants that support cognitive function and heart health.
- Honey: A natural sweetener that adds sweetness without spiking blood sugar levels.

This Roasted Beet and Citrus Salad is a flavorful and nutrient-rich option for seniors. It combines the brain-boosting properties of beets and citrus fruits with the creaminess of goat cheese and the crunch of nuts. The dressing adds a touch of sweetness and tang, making it a wholesome addition to your meals.

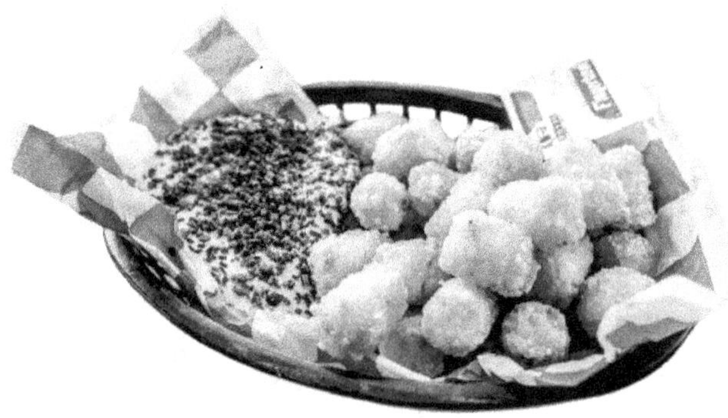

Quinoa and Avocado Salad

Time of Preparation: 20 minutes

Ingredients:

For the Salad:
- 1 cup quinoa, rinsed
- 2 cups water
- 1 large avocado, diced
- 1 cup cherry tomatoes, halved
- 1/4 cup red onion, finely chopped
- 1/4 cup cucumber, diced
- 1/4 cup fresh cilantro, chopped
- 1/4 cup crumbled feta cheese (optional)
- Salt and pepper to taste

For the Dressing:
- 2 tablespoons extra-virgin olive oil
- 1 tablespoon lemon juice
- 1 teaspoon honey (optional for sweetness)
- 1/2 teaspoon cumin (optional)
- Salt and pepper to taste

Method of Preparation:
1. Put the quinoa and water in a medium-sized pot. After bringing it to a boil, lower the heat to a simmer, cover it, and cook the quinoa for approximately fifteen minutes, or until it is tender and the liquid has been absorbed.
2. Fluff the cooked quinoa with a fork and let it cool.

3. In a large salad bowl, combine the cooked quinoa, diced avocado, cherry tomatoes, chopped red onion, diced cucumber, and chopped cilantro. If desired, add crumbled feta cheese.

4. In a separate small bowl, whisk together the extra-virgin olive oil, lemon juice, honey (if using), cumin (if using), salt, and pepper to create the dressing.

5. Drizzle the dressing over the salad and toss to combine.

6. Serve immediately.

Nutritional Benefits for Seniors:

- Quinoa: A source of protein, fiber, vitamins, and minerals that support cognitive health and overall well-being.

- Avocado: Rich in healthy monounsaturated fats, vitamin E, and antioxidants that promote brain and heart health.

- Cherry Tomatoes: Provide antioxidants, vitamins, and minerals that protect brain cells and promote cognitive function.

- Red Onion: Contains antioxidants and anti-inflammatory compounds that may support cognitive health.

- Cucumber: Low in calories and provides hydration, contributing to overall well-being.

- Cilantro: A source of antioxidants and vitamins that support brain health.

- Feta Cheese (Optional): Adds calcium and protein, essential for bone and muscle health in seniors.

- Olive Oil: Contains monounsaturated fats and antioxidants that support cognitive function and heart health.
- Honey (Optional): A natural sweetener that adds sweetness without spiking blood sugar levels.

This Quinoa and Avocado Salad is a nutritious and satisfying choice for seniors. It combines the brain-boosting properties of quinoa and avocado with the freshness of vegetables and a flavorful dressing. It's a wholesome addition to your meals.

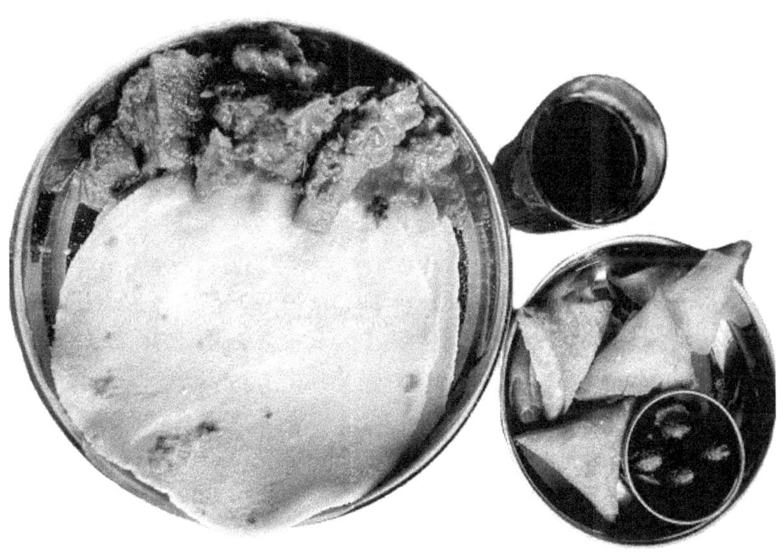

Hummus and Veggie Platter

Time of Preparation: 15 minutes

Ingredients:

For the Hummus:
-One can (15 ounces) of rinsed and drained chickpeas
- 2 tablespoons tahini
- 2 tablespoons lemon juice
- 1-2 cloves garlic, minced
- 2 tablespoons extra-virgin olive oil
- 1/2 teaspoon ground cumin
- Salt and pepper to taste
- Water (for desired consistency)

For the Veggie Platter:
- An assortment of fresh vegetables such as baby carrots, cucumber slices, bell pepper strips, cherry tomatoes, celery sticks, and broccoli florets
- Optional fresh herb garnish, such as cilantro or parsley

Method of Preparation:

For the Hummus:
1. In a food processor, combine the chickpeas, tahini, lemon juice, minced garlic, extra-virgin olive oil, ground cumin, salt, and pepper.

2. Process the ingredients until smooth. To get the right consistency, thin up any excess hummus by adding a little amount of water.
3. Taste and adjust the seasonings, adding more lemon juice, garlic, salt, or pepper if needed.
4. Transfer the hummus to a serving bowl and drizzle with a bit of extra-virgin olive oil.
5. Optionally, garnish with fresh herbs.

For the Veggie Platter:
1. Wash and prepare the assortment of fresh vegetables by cutting them into bite-sized pieces or sticks.
2. Arrange the prepared vegetables around the bowl of hummus on a serving platter.
3. Serve immediately.

Nutritional Benefits for Seniors:
- Chickpeas (Hummus): Rich in protein, fiber, and nutrients that support brain health and overall well-being.
- Tahini (Hummus): A source of healthy fats, vitamins, and minerals that promote brain and heart health.
- Lemon Juice (Hummus): Provides vitamin C and citrus bioflavonoids that protect brain cells and promote cognitive function.
- Fresh Vegetables: Offer a variety of vitamins, minerals, and antioxidants that support brain health and overall well-being.
- Extra-Virgin Olive Oil (Hummus): Contains monounsaturated fats and antioxidants that support cognitive function and heart health.

This Hummus and Veggie Platter is a delightful and nutritious snack or appetizer for seniors. It combines the protein-packed goodness of hummus with a colorful assortment of fresh vegetables. It's a delicious and healthful option for any occasion.

Superfood Avocado Bruschetta

Time of Preparation: 15 minutes

Ingredients:

For the Avocado Topping:
- 2 ripe avocados, diced
- 1/2 cup cherry tomatoes, diced
- 1/4 cup red onion, finely chopped
- 2 teaspoons chopped fresh parsley or cilantro.
- 1 tablespoon extra-virgin olive oil
- 1 tablespoon lemon juice
- Salt and pepper to taste

For the Bruschetta Base:
- Baguette or whole-grain bread, sliced
- 1 clove garlic, peeled
- Olive oil for toasting

Method of Preparation:

For the Avocado Topping:

1. In a bowl, combine the diced avocados, diced cherry tomatoes, finely chopped red onion, chopped cilantro or parsley, extra-virgin olive oil, lemon juice, salt, and pepper.
2. Gently toss the ingredients until well combined.
3. Taste and adjust the seasonings, adding more lemon juice, salt, or pepper if needed.

For the Bruschetta Base:
1. Preheat your oven's broiler or a toaster.
2. Place the bread slices under the broiler or in the toaster and toast them until they are lightly browned on both sides.
3. While the bread is still warm, rub one side of each slice with the peeled garlic clove. This imparts a subtle garlic flavor.
4. Drizzle a little olive oil over the garlic-rubbed side of each toast.

To Serve:
1. Arrange the toasted bruschetta slices on a serving platter with the garlic-rubbed side facing up.
2. Spoon the avocado topping generously onto each slice.
3. Serve immediately.

Nutritional Benefits for Seniors:
- Avocado: Rich in healthy monounsaturated fats, vitamin E, and antioxidants that promote brain and heart health.

- Cherry Tomatoes: Provide antioxidants, vitamins, and minerals that protect brain cells and promote cognitive function.
- Red Onion: Contains antioxidants and anti-inflammatory compounds that may support cognitive health.
- Fresh Herbs (Cilantro or Parsley): A source of antioxidants and vitamins that support brain health.
- Olive Oil: Contains monounsaturated fats and antioxidants that support cognitive function and heart health.
- Whole-Grain Bread: Provides complex carbohydrates and fiber for sustained energy and digestive health.

This Superfood Avocado Bruschetta is a delicious and nutrient-rich appetizer or snack for seniors. It combines the creamy goodness of avocado with the freshness of cherry tomatoes and the flavors of garlic and herbs, all served on toasted whole-grain bread. It's a superfood-packed treat for any occasion.

Chapter 4: Main Courses

Baked Salmon with Lemon-Dill Sauce

Time of Preparation: 30 minutes

Ingredients:

For the Baked Salmon:
-Four salmon fillets, each weighing around six ounces
- 2 tablespoons olive oil
- 2 cloves garlic, minced
- 1 tablespoon or 1 teaspoon of chopped fresh dill.
- Salt and pepper to taste
- Lemon slices for garnish

For the Lemon-Dill Sauce:
- 1/2 cup plain Greek yogurt
- 1 tablespoon fresh lemon juice
- 1 tablespoon fresh dill, chopped
- 1 teaspoon honey (optional for sweetness)
- Salt and pepper to taste

Method of Preparation:

For the Baked Salmon:
1. Preheat your oven to 375°F (190°C).
2. Transfer the salmon fillets to a parchment paper-lined baking sheet.

3. In a small bowl, combine the olive oil, minced garlic, dried or fresh dill, salt, and pepper.
4. Brush the salmon fillets with the olive oil mixture, ensuring they are evenly coated.
5. Place a lemon slice on top of each fillet.
6. Bake in the preheated oven for about 15-20 minutes, or until the salmon flakes easily with a fork.

For the Lemon-Dill Sauce:
1. In a small bowl, combine the plain Greek yogurt, fresh lemon juice, fresh dill, honey (if using), salt, and pepper.
2. Mix the ingredients until smooth.

To Serve:
1. Drizzle the lemon-dill sauce over the baked salmon fillets.
2. Garnish with additional fresh dill and lemon slices.
3. Serve immediately.

Nutritional Benefits for Seniors:
- Salmon: A source of omega-3 fatty acids and high-quality protein that are essential for cognitive and heart health.
- Olive Oil: Contains monounsaturated fats and antioxidants that support cognitive function and heart health.
- Garlic: Provides anti-inflammatory properties that may benefit cognitive health.
- Dill: An herb with potential anti-inflammatory and antioxidant properties.

- Greek Yogurt (Lemon-Dill Sauce): Offers protein, probiotics, and calcium, essential for muscle, digestive, and bone health.
- Lemon: Provides vitamin C and citrus bioflavonoids that protect brain cells and promote cognitive function.
- Honey (Optional): A natural sweetener that adds sweetness without spiking blood sugar levels.

This Baked Salmon with Lemon-Dill Sauce is a flavorful and nutritious main course for seniors. It combines the heart-healthy benefits of salmon with the freshness of dill and the zing of lemon in the sauce. It's a delightful and brain-boosting addition to your meals.

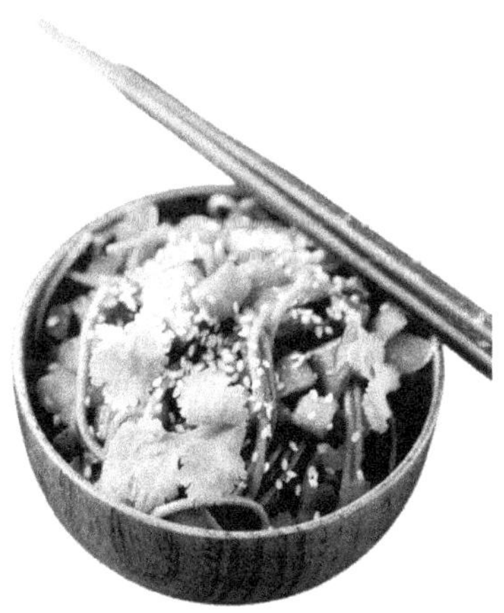

Grilled Mackerel with Herbed Quinoa

Time of Preparation: 30 minutes

Ingredients:

For the Grilled Mackerel:
-Four mackerel fillets, weighing almost six ounces each
- 2 tablespoons olive oil
- 2 cloves garlic, minced
- 1 teaspoon dried oregano
- 1 teaspoon dried thyme
- Salt and pepper to taste
- Lemon wedges for garnish

For the Herbed Quinoa:
- 1 cup quinoa, rinsed
- 2 cups water or vegetable broth
- 2 tablespoons fresh parsley, chopped
- 2 tablespoons fresh dill, chopped
- 1 tablespoon fresh lemon juice
- Salt and pepper to taste

Method of Preparation:

For the Grilled Mackerel:
1. Preheat your grill to medium-high heat.
2. In a small bowl, combine the olive oil, minced garlic, dried oregano, dried thyme, salt, and pepper.

3. Brush the mackerel fillets with the olive oil mixture, ensuring they are evenly coated.

4. Place the mackerel fillets on the preheated grill and cook for about 4-5 minutes per side or until the fish flakes easily with a fork.

5. Remove the grilled mackerel from the heat and keep warm.

For the Herbed Quinoa:

1. In a medium saucepan, combine the quinoa and water or vegetable broth. After bringing it to a boil, lower the heat to a simmer, cover it, and cook the quinoa for approximately fifteen minutes, or until it is tender and the liquid has been absorbed.

2. Fluff the cooked quinoa with a fork.

3. Stir in the fresh parsley, fresh dill, fresh lemon juice, salt, and pepper.

To Serve:

1. Divide the herbed quinoa among serving plates.

2. Place the grilled mackerel fillets on top of the quinoa.

3. Garnish with lemon wedges.

4. Serve immediately.

Nutritional Benefits for Seniors:

- Mackerel: A fatty fish rich in omega-3 fatty acids and high-quality protein that are essential for cognitive and heart health.

- Olive Oil (Grilled Mackerel): Contains monounsaturated fats and antioxidants that support cognitive function and heart health.

- Oregano and Thyme (Grilled Mackerel): Herbs with potential anti-inflammatory and antioxidant properties.
- Quinoa (Herbed Quinoa): A source of protein, fiber, vitamins, and minerals that support cognitive health and overall well-being.
- Parsley and Dill (Herbed Quinoa): Herbs with antioxidants and vitamins that support brain health.
- Lemon (Herbed Quinoa): Provides vitamin C and citrus bioflavonoids that protect brain cells and promote cognitive function.

This Grilled Mackerel with Herbed Quinoa is a flavorful and nutritious main course for seniors. It combines the brain-boosting benefits of mackerel with the freshness of herbs and lemon-infused quinoa. It's a delicious and wholesome addition to your meals.

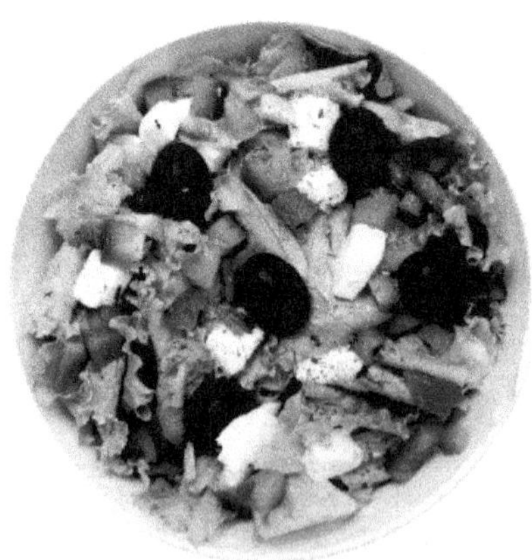

Lentil and Vegetable Stir-Fry

Time of Preparation: 30 minutes

Ingredients:

For the Lentil Stir-Fry:
- 1 cup of dry lentils, washed and drained, either brown or green
- 2 cups vegetable broth or water
- 2 tablespoons olive oil
- 1 onion, chopped
- 2 cloves garlic, minced
- 2 carrots, sliced
- 1 red bell pepper, sliced
- 1 zucchini, sliced
- 1 cup broccoli florets
- 1 cup snow peas
- 1/4 cup low-sodium soy sauce
- 1 tablespoon honey (optional for sweetness)
- 1 teaspoon ground ginger
- Salt and pepper to taste

Method of Preparation:

For the Lentil Stir-Fry:
1. In a medium saucepan, combine the lentils and vegetable broth or water. Bring it to a boil, then reduce the heat to low, cover, and simmer for about 20-25 minutes or until the lentils are tender but still firm.

2. Drain any excess liquid from the cooked lentils.

3. In a large wok or skillet, heat the olive oil over medium-high heat.

4. Add the chopped onion and minced garlic and sauté for 2-3 minutes until they are softened.

5. Add the sliced carrots, red bell pepper, zucchini, broccoli florets, and snow peas. Stir-fry for about 5-7 minutes or until the vegetables are crisp-tender.

6. In a small bowl, combine the low-sodium soy sauce, honey (if using), ground ginger, salt, and pepper.

7. Pour the sauce over the vegetables and stir to combine.

8. Add the cooked lentils to the stir-fry and gently toss until everything is heated through.

Nutritional Benefits for Seniors:
- Lentils: Rich in fiber, protein, vitamins, and minerals that support cognitive health and overall well-being.
- Vegetables (Carrots, Red Bell Pepper, Zucchini, Broccoli, Snow Peas): Provide a variety of vitamins, minerals, and antioxidants that protect brain cells and promote cognitive function.
- Olive Oil: Contains monounsaturated fats and antioxidants that support cognitive function and heart health.
- Soy Sauce: Adds flavor and provides amino acids for cognitive function.

This Lentil and Vegetable Stir-Fry is a hearty and nutritious meal for seniors. It combines the brain-boosting benefits of lentils with an array of colorful and fresh vegetables. The stir-fry is seasoned with a flavorful sauce that enhances the overall taste. It's a satisfying and wholesome addition to your meals.

Spaghetti Squash with Pesto

Time of Preparation: 45 minutes

Ingredients:

For the Spaghetti Squash:
- 1 spaghetti squash
- 2 tablespoons olive oil
- Salt and pepper to taste

For the Pesto:
- 2 cups fresh basil leaves
- 1/2 cup grated Parmesan cheese
- 1/2 cup pine nuts
- 2 cloves garlic
- 1/2 cup extra-virgin olive oil
- 1 tablespoon lemon juice
- Salt and pepper to taste

Method of Preparation:

For the Spaghetti Squash:
1. Preheat your oven to 375°F (190°C).
2. Cut the spaghetti squash in half lengthwise and remove the seeds and stringy bits with a spoon.

3. Brush the cut sides of the squash with olive oil and season with salt and pepper.

4. On a baking sheet covered with parchment paper, arrange the squash halves cut-side down.

5. Bake in the preheated oven for about 30-40 minutes or until the squash is tender and the flesh can be easily shredded with a fork.

6. Remove the squash from the oven and let it cool slightly.

7. Use a fork to scrape the flesh of the squash, creating "spaghetti" strands.

For the Pesto:

1. Put the garlic, pine nuts, grated Parmesan cheese, and fresh basil leaves in a food processor.

2. Pulse the ingredients until finely chopped.

3. With the food processor running, slowly drizzle in the extra-virgin olive oil until the pesto is well blended.

4. Add the lemon juice, salt, and pepper, and pulse to combine.

To Serve:

1. Divide the spaghetti squash strands among serving plates.

2. Drizzle the pesto over the spaghetti squash.

3. Toss to combine and coat the squash with the pesto.

4. Serve immediately.

Nutritional Benefits for Seniors:

- Spaghetti Squash: A low-calorie, low-carb alternative to pasta that provides vitamins, minerals, and dietary fiber for brain and digestive health.
- Olive Oil (Pesto): Contains monounsaturated fats and antioxidants that support cognitive function and heart health.
- Basil (Pesto): An herb with antioxidants and potential anti-inflammatory properties that support brain health.
- Parmesan Cheese (Pesto): Adds flavor and provides protein and calcium for cognitive and bone health.
- Pine Nuts (Pesto): Offer healthy fats, protein, and minerals that may promote cognitive function.

This Spaghetti Squash with Pesto is a light and flavorful dish for seniors. It combines the texture of spaghetti squash with the rich taste of homemade basil pesto. The result is a satisfying and brain-boosting meal that's both delicious and nutritious.

Chicken and Spanish Stuffed Bell Peppers

Time of Preparation: 1 hour

Ingredients:

For the Stuffed Bell Peppers:
- 4 big bell peppers (any colour), seeded and with the tops removed
- 1 pound ground chicken
- 1 small onion, finely chopped
- 2 cloves garlic, minced
- 1 cup cooked brown rice
- 1 can (15 ounces) diced tomatoes
- 1 teaspoon ground cumin
- 1/2 teaspoon paprika
- Salt and pepper to taste

For Topping:
- 1/2 cup shredded cheddar cheese
- Fresh cilantro for garnish (optional)

Method of Preparation:

For the Stuffed Bell Peppers:
1. Preheat your oven to 375°F (190°C).

2. In a large skillet, cook the ground chicken over medium heat until it's no longer pink. Break it into small pieces as it cooks.

3. Add the chopped onion and minced garlic to the skillet and sauté until they are softened.

4. Stir in the cooked brown rice, diced tomatoes, ground cumin, paprika, salt, and pepper. Mix well and cook for a few more minutes until the mixture is heated through.

5. Carefully stuff the bell peppers with the chicken and rice mixture.

6. Transfer the filled bell peppers to a baking plate.

7. Cover the dish with aluminum foil.

8. Bake in the preheated oven for about 30-40 minutes or until the peppers are tender.

9. Remove the foil, sprinkle the shredded cheddar cheese on top of each stuffed pepper, and return to the oven for a few minutes until the cheese is melted and bubbly.

10. Garnish with fresh cilantro if desired.

Nutritional Benefits for Seniors:

- Bell Peppers: Provide vitamins, minerals, and antioxidants that support brain health and overall well-being.

- Ground Chicken: A source of protein and essential nutrients that are important for cognitive and muscle health.

- Onion: Contains antioxidants and anti-inflammatory compounds that may support cognitive health.

- Garlic: Provides anti-inflammatory properties that may benefit cognitive health.

- Brown Rice: Offers complex carbohydrates, fiber, and vitamins that support cognitive function and digestive health.
- Diced Tomatoes: Rich in vitamins, minerals, and antioxidants that protect brain cells and promote cognitive function.
- Cheddar Cheese: Adds flavor and provides protein and calcium for cognitive and bone health.
- Cumin and Paprika: Spices that can add flavor and potential health benefits.

This Chicken and Spanish Stuffed Bell Peppers recipe is a wholesome and satisfying meal for seniors. It combines the flavors of chicken, rice, and tomatoes inside tender bell peppers, all topped with melted cheddar cheese. It's a delicious and nutritious dish that's sure to be enjoyed.

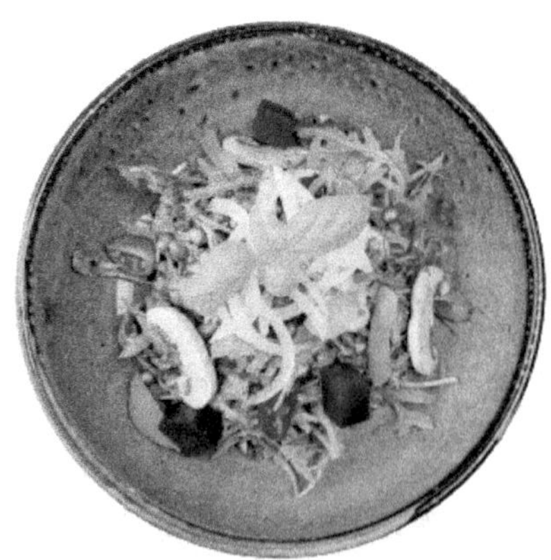

Chapter 5: Sides and Snacks

Broccoli and Cheddar Stuffed Potatoes

Time of Preparation: 1 hour

Ingredients:

For the Stuffed Potatoes:
- 4 large russet potatoes
- 2 cups broccoli florets, steamed and chopped
- 1 cup shredded cheddar cheese
- 1/2 cup plain Greek yogurt
- 2 tablespoons butter
- Salt and pepper to taste

For Topping:
- Garnish with chopped green onions or chives (optional)

Method of Preparation:

For the Stuffed Potatoes:
1. Preheat your oven to 400°F (200°C).
2. Scrub the russet potatoes and pierce them with a fork in several places.
3. Place the potatoes on a baking sheet and bake in the preheated oven for about 45-60 minutes, or until they are tender when pierced with a fork.

4. While the potatoes are baking, steam the broccoli florets until they are tender. Then, chop them into small pieces.

5. Take the potatoes out of the oven when they are done and allow them to cool slightly.

6. Cut off the top third of each potato and scoop out the flesh, leaving a thin shell.

7. In a mixing bowl, combine the scooped-out potato flesh, chopped broccoli, shredded cheddar cheese, plain Greek yogurt, and butter.

8. Mash and mix the ingredients together until well combined. Season with salt and pepper.

9. Stuff the potato shells with the broccoli and cheddar mixture.

10. Return the stuffed potatoes to the oven and bake for an additional 10-15 minutes, or until the filling is heated through and the tops are slightly golden.

11. Garnish with chopped chives or green onions if desired.

Nutritional Benefits for Seniors:
- Potatoes: A source of carbohydrates, fiber, vitamins, and minerals that provide energy and support cognitive function.
- Broccoli: Rich in vitamins, minerals, and antioxidants that protect brain cells and promote cognitive function.
- Cheddar Cheese: Adds flavor and provides protein and calcium for cognitive and bone health.
- Greek Yogurt: Offers protein, probiotics, and calcium, essential for muscle, digestive, and bone health.
- Butter: Provides healthy fats and flavor.

- Chives or Green Onions (Optional): Herbs that add flavor and potential health benefits.

These Broccoli and Cheddar Stuffed Potatoes are a comforting and nutritious dish for seniors. They combine the heartiness of russet potatoes with the goodness of broccoli and cheddar cheese. The Greek yogurt adds creaminess, making it a delightful addition to your meals.

Roasted Sweet Potato Fries

Time of Preparation: 30 minutes

Ingredients:

- Two big sweet potatoes, sliced into fries after peeling.
- 2 tablespoons olive oil
- 1 teaspoon paprika
- 1/2 teaspoon garlic powder
- 1/2 teaspoon onion powder
- Salt and pepper to taste
- Fresh parsley for garnish (optional)

Method of Preparation:

1. Preheat your oven to 425°F (220°C).
2. In a large mixing bowl, combine the sweet potato fries, olive oil, paprika, garlic powder, onion powder, salt,

and pepper. Toss to coat the fries evenly with the seasonings and oil.
3. Spread the seasoned sweet potato fries in a single layer on a baking sheet lined with parchment paper.
4. Bake in the preheated oven for about 20-25 minutes, turning them halfway through, or until the fries are crispy and browned.
5. Remove the roasted sweet potato fries from the oven.
6. Garnish with fresh parsley if desired.
7. Serve immediately.

Nutritional Benefits for Seniors:
- Sweet Potatoes: A source of complex carbohydrates, fiber, vitamins, and minerals that support cognitive health and provide energy.
- Olive Oil: Contains monounsaturated fats and antioxidants that support cognitive function and heart health.
- Paprika, Garlic Powder, and Onion Powder: Spices that add flavor and potential health benefits.

These Roasted Sweet Potato Fries are a tasty and nutritious side dish for seniors. They combine the natural sweetness of sweet potatoes with a blend of spices, creating a satisfying and crispy texture. It's a delightful addition to your meals, and they make a healthy alternative to traditional fries.

Walnut and Rosemary Crackers

Time of Preparation: 45 minutes

Ingredients:

- 1 cup all-purpose flour
- 1/2 cup whole wheat flour
- 1/2 cup chopped walnuts
- 1 tablespoon fresh rosemary, finely chopped
- 1/2 teaspoon salt
- 1/4 teaspoon black pepper
- 1/4 cup olive oil
- 1/2 cup water

Method of Preparation:

1. Preheat your oven to 375°F (190°C).
2. In a mixing bowl, combine the all-purpose flour, whole wheat flour, chopped walnuts, finely chopped fresh rosemary, salt, and black pepper.
3. Add the olive oil and water to the dry ingredients and mix until a dough forms. It could be necessary to slightly modify the water quantity in order to attain the desired consistency.
4. Cut the dough in half, equally.

5. Roll out each portion of dough on a lightly floured surface to your desired thickness, usually about 1/8 inch thick.

6. Use a cookie cutter or a knife to cut the rolled-out dough into cracker-sized pieces or any shape you prefer.

7. Transfer the cut crackers to a baking sheet lined with parchment paper, leaving some space between them.

8. Bake in the preheated oven for about 15-20 minutes or until the crackers are golden brown and crisp.

9. Remove the walnut and rosemary crackers from the oven and let them cool on a wire rack.

10. Once cooled, store the crackers in an airtight container.

Nutritional Benefits for Seniors:
- Walnuts: A source of omega-3 fatty acids, antioxidants, and essential nutrients that support cognitive and heart health.
- Rosemary: An herb with potential cognitive and anti-inflammatory benefits.

These Walnut and Rosemary Crackers are a flavorful and nutrient-rich snack for seniors. They combine the earthy taste of whole wheat flour with the richness of walnuts and the aromatic touch of fresh rosemary. These homemade crackers are perfect for enjoying with dips or on their own.

Kale Chips with Parmesan

Time of Preparation: 20 minutes

Ingredients:

- 1 bunch of fresh kale, washed and dried
- 2 tablespoons olive oil
- 1/4 cup grated Parmesan cheese
- Salt and pepper to taste

Method of Preparation:

1. Preheat your oven to 300°F (150°C).
2. Remove the tough stems from the kale leaves, and tear the leaves into bite-sized pieces.
3. In a large mixing bowl, drizzle the torn kale leaves with olive oil and toss to coat evenly.
4. Arrange the kale pieces in a single layer on a baking sheet lined with parchment paper.
5. Sprinkle the grated Parmesan cheese over the kale leaves.
6. Add a little salt and a little pepper for seasoning.
7. Bake in the preheated oven for about 12-15 minutes or until the kale is crispy and the cheese is golden brown.
8. Remove the kale chips from the oven and let them cool on the baking sheet.
9. Serve immediately.

Nutritional Benefits for Seniors:
- Kale: A leafy green vegetable packed with vitamins, minerals, antioxidants, and fiber that support brain health and overall well-being.
- Olive Oil: Contains monounsaturated fats and antioxidants that support cognitive function and heart health.
- Parmesan Cheese: Adds flavor and provides protein and calcium for cognitive and bone health.

These Kale Chips with Parmesan are a delicious and nutritious snack for seniors. They transform fresh kale into crispy chips with a delightful cheesy flavor. They make for a satisfying and wholesome treat that's perfect for munching on any time.

Edamame with Sea Salt

Time of Preparation: 10 minutes

Ingredients:

- 2 cups frozen edamame (young soybeans)
- Sea salt, to taste

Method of Preparation:

1. Start by boiling a kettle of water.
2. Put the frozen edamame into the water that is boiling.

3. Cook for about 4-5 minutes, or until the edamame is tender.
4. Drain the cooked edamame.
5. Sprinkle it with sea salt while they are still hot.
6. Toss to coat evenly.
7. Serve immediately.

Nutritional Benefits for Seniors:
- Edamame: A good source of plant-based protein, fiber, vitamins, and minerals that support cognitive health and overall well-being.

These Edamame with Sea Salt are a simple, quick, and nutritious snack for seniors. Edamame provides plant-based protein and fiber and can be enjoyed with a sprinkle of sea salt for added flavor. They make a wholesome and satisfying option for anytime snacking.

Chapter 6: Soups and Stews

Tomato and Basil Soup

Time of Preparation: 30 minutes

Ingredients:

- 1 can (28 ounces) whole tomatoes
- 1 tablespoon olive oil
- 1 onion, chopped
- 2 cloves garlic, minced
- 1/4 cup fresh basil leaves, chopped
- 4 cups vegetable broth
- Salt and pepper to taste
- 1/2 cup heavy cream (optional)
- Fresh basil leaves for garnish (optional)

Method of Preparation:

1. Place the olive oil in a big saucepan and heat it to medium.
2. Add the chopped onion and minced garlic, and sauté until they are softened and fragrant.
3. Add the whole tomatoes to the pot, breaking them up with a spoon.
4. Stir in the fresh basil leaves.
5. After adding the vegetable broth, boil the mixture.
6. To taste, add salt and pepper for seasoning.

7. Simmer for about 15-20 minutes, allowing the flavors to meld together.

8. If desired, use an immersion blender to puree the soup until smooth. Alternatively, transfer the soup in batches to a regular blender and blend until smooth. In a blender, use hot liquids with caution.

9. Return the blended soup to the pot and heat through.

10. If using, stir in the heavy cream to add a creamy texture.

11. Taste and adjust the seasoning if needed.

12. Serve hot, garnished with fresh basil leaves if desired.

Nutritional Benefits for Seniors:

- Tomatoes: A source of antioxidants, vitamins, and minerals that protect brain cells and promote cognitive function.

- Olive Oil: Contains monounsaturated fats and antioxidants that support cognitive function and heart health.

- Basil: An herb with antioxidants and potential anti-inflammatory properties that support brain health.

- Heavy Cream (Optional): Adds richness and flavor to the soup.

This Tomato and Basil Soup is a comforting and nutrient-rich option for seniors. It combines the rich flavor of tomatoes with the freshness of basil, creating a soothing and aromatic soup. The optional addition of heavy cream makes it even more velvety. It's a perfect choice for a warm and satisfying meal.

<u>Vegetable and Bean Minestrone</u>

Time of Preparation: 45 minutes

Ingredients:

- 2 tablespoons olive oil
- 1 onion, chopped
- 2 cloves garlic, minced
- 1 carrot, diced
- 1 celery stalk, diced
- 1 zucchini, diced
- 1 yellow squash, diced
-Rinse and drain 15 ounces of canned kidney beans.
-Scoop out and rinse one can (15 ounces) of cannellini beans.
- 1 can (15 ounces) diced tomatoes
- 4 cups vegetable broth
- 1 teaspoon dried oregano
- 1 teaspoon dried basil
- Salt and pepper to taste
- 1 cup small pasta (e.g., ditalini or small shells)
- Fresh parsley for garnish (optional)
- Grated Parmesan cheese for garnish (optional)

Method of Preparation:

1. Place the olive oil in a big saucepan and heat it to medium.

2. Add the chopped onion and minced garlic, and sauté until they are softened and fragrant.

3. Add the diced carrot, celery, zucchini, and yellow squash. Sauté for a few minutes until the vegetables start to soften.

4. Stir in the kidney beans, cannellini beans, diced tomatoes, vegetable broth, dried oregano, dried basil, salt, and pepper.

5. Allow the mixture to boil for 15 to 20 minutes at a simmer so that the flavors may combine.

6. While the soup is simmering, cook the small pasta separately according to the package instructions. Drain and set aside.

7. Once the soup is ready, stir in the cooked pasta.

8. Taste and, if necessary, adjust the seasoning.

9. Serve hot, garnished with fresh parsley and grated Parmesan cheese if desired.

Nutritional Benefits for Seniors:

- Beans (Kidney and Cannellini): A source of plant-based protein, fiber, vitamins, and minerals that support cognitive health and overall well-being.

- Vegetables (Carrot, Celery, Zucchini, Yellow Squash): Provide a variety of vitamins, minerals, and antioxidants that protect brain cells and promote cognitive function.

- Diced Tomatoes: Rich in vitamins, minerals, and antioxidants that protect brain cells and promote cognitive function.

- Olive Oil: Contains monounsaturated fats and antioxidants that support cognitive function and heart health.

- Pasta: Offers carbohydrates for energy and dietary fiber for digestive health.
- Dried Oregano and Basil: Spices that add flavor and potential health benefits.

This Vegetable and Bean Minestrone is a hearty and wholesome soup for seniors. It's filled with an assortment of beans, vegetables, and pasta, all simmered in a savory broth with herbs and spices. It's a satisfying and nutritious choice for a comforting meal.

Chicken and Vegetable Stew

Time of Preparation: 1 hour

Ingredients:

- Four skinless, boneless chicken thighs, diced into small pieces
- 2 tablespoons olive oil
- 1 onion, chopped
- 2 cloves garlic, minced
- 1 carrot, sliced
- 1 celery stalk, sliced
- 1 zucchini, diced
- 1 yellow squash, diced
- 1 can (15 ounces) diced tomatoes
- 4 cups chicken broth
- 1 teaspoon dried thyme

- 1 teaspoon dried rosemary
- Salt and pepper to taste
- One cup of finely chopped and bite-sized green beans
- Fresh parsley for garnish (optional)

Method of Preparation:

1. Place the olive oil in a big saucepan and heat it to medium.
2. Add the chopped onion and minced garlic, and sauté until they are softened and fragrant.
3. Include the chicken pieces and cook them through, browning all over.
4. Stir in the sliced carrot, celery, zucchini, and yellow squash. Sauté for a few minutes until the vegetables start to soften.
5. Add the diced tomatoes, chicken broth, dried thyme, dried rosemary, salt, and pepper.
6. Bring the mixture to a simmer and let it cook for about 30-40 minutes, allowing the flavors to meld together.
7. About 10 minutes before serving, stir in the green beans and let them cook until tender.
8. Taste and, if necessary, adjust the seasoning.
9. If preferred, garnished with freshly chopped parsley and serve hot.

Nutritional Benefits for Seniors:
- Chicken: A source of protein and essential nutrients that are important for cognitive and muscle health.
- Vegetables (Carrot, Celery, Zucchini, Yellow Squash, Green Beans): Provide a variety of vitamins, minerals,

and antioxidants that protect brain cells and promote cognitive function.
- Diced Tomatoes: Rich in vitamins, minerals, and antioxidants that protect brain cells and promote cognitive function.
- Olive Oil: Contains monounsaturated fats and antioxidants that support cognitive function and heart health.
- Dried Thyme and Rosemary: Herbs that add flavor and potential health benefits.

This Chicken and Vegetable Stew is a wholesome and satisfying meal for seniors. It combines tender chicken pieces with a medley of colorful vegetables in a flavorful broth. The herbs and spices add a delightful touch to this comforting stew. It's perfect for nourishing and warming the body.

Butternut Squash and Sage Soup

Time of Preparation: 45 minutes

Ingredients:

-A single butternut squash, chopped, skinned, and seeded
- 2 tablespoons olive oil
- 1 onion, chopped
- 2 cloves garlic, minced
- 1 carrot, sliced

- 1 celery stalk, sliced
- 1 potato, peeled and diced
- 4 cups vegetable broth
- 1 teaspoon dried sage
- Salt and pepper to taste
- 1/2 cup heavy cream (optional)
- Fresh sage leaves for garnish (optional)

Method of Preparation:

1. Place the olive oil in a big saucepan and heat it to medium.
2. Add the chopped onion and minced garlic, and sauté until they are softened and fragrant.
3. Stir in the diced butternut squash, carrot, celery, and potato. Sauté for a few minutes until the vegetables start to soften.
4. Pour in the vegetable broth, dried sage, salt, and pepper.
5. Bring the mixture to a simmer and let it cook for about 25-30 minutes, or until the vegetables are tender.
6. Using an immersion blender, puree the soup until smooth. Alternatively, transfer the soup in batches to a regular blender and blend until smooth. In a blender, use hot liquids with caution.
7. Return the blended soup to the pot and heat through.
8. If using, stir in the heavy cream to add a creamy texture.
9. Taste and, if necessary, adjust the seasoning.
10. Serve hot, garnished with fresh sage leaves if desired.

Nutritional Benefits for Seniors:
- Butternut Squash: A source of vitamins, minerals, and antioxidants that support brain health and overall well-being.
- Vegetables (Carrot, Celery, Potato): Provide a variety of vitamins, minerals, and antioxidants that protect brain cells and promote cognitive function.
- Olive Oil: Contains monounsaturated fats and antioxidants that support cognitive function and heart health.
- Sage (Dried and Fresh): An herb with antioxidants and potential cognitive benefits.
- Heavy Cream (Optional): Adds richness and flavor to the soup.

This Butternut Squash and Sage Soup is a comforting and nutrient-rich choice for seniors. It combines the sweetness of butternut squash with the earthy flavor of sage, creating a smooth and velvety soup. The optional addition of heavy cream makes it even more luscious. It's a perfect option for a warm and nourishing meal.

Chapter 7: Desserts

Dark Chocolate and Berry Parfait

Time of Preparation: 15 minutes

Ingredients:

- 1 cup low-fat Greek yogurt
- 2 tablespoons dark chocolate chips
- 1 cup mixed berries (e.g., strawberries, blueberries, raspberries)
- 1 tablespoon honey
- 2 tablespoons granola
- Fresh mint leaves for garnish (optional)

Method of Preparation:

1. In a small microwave-safe bowl, melt the dark chocolate chips in the microwave in 20-second increments until smooth. Stir well.
2. In a serving glass or bowl, start by layering 1/4 cup of low-fat Greek yogurt.
3. Add a drizzle of the melted dark chocolate over the yogurt.
4. Add a layer of mixed berries.
5. Repeat the layers until you've used all the ingredients, finishing with a layer of berries on top.
6. Drizzle honey over the berry layer.

7. Sprinkle granola over the honey.
8. If you'd like, garnish with freshly chopped mint leaves.
9. Serve immediately.

Nutritional Benefits for Seniors:
- Greek Yogurt: A source of protein, probiotics, and calcium, essential for muscle, digestive, and bone health.
- Dark Chocolate: Provides antioxidants and potential cognitive and heart health benefits.
- Berries (Strawberries, Blueberries, Raspberries): Rich in vitamins, minerals, and antioxidants that protect brain cells and promote cognitive function.
- Honey: Adds natural sweetness and potential anti-inflammatory properties.
- Granola: Offers whole grains and fiber for energy and digestive health.

This Dark Chocolate and Berry Parfait is a delightful and nutritious dessert for seniors. It combines the creaminess of Greek yogurt with the richness of dark chocolate and the freshness of mixed berries. The honey drizzle and granola add a sweet and crunchy touch. It's the ideal option for a guilt-free indulgence.

Almond and Blueberry Bites

Time of Preparation: 15 minutes

Ingredients:

- 1 cup whole almonds
- 1/2 cup dried blueberries
- 1/4 cup honey
- 1/4 cup almond butter
- 1 teaspoon vanilla extract
- 1/2 teaspoon ground cinnamon
- 1/4 teaspoon salt
- 1/2 cup unsweetened shredded coconut (for coating)

Method of Preparation:

1. In a food processor, combine the whole almonds and dried blueberries. Pulse until they are finely chopped.
2. In a mixing bowl, combine the chopped almond and blueberry mixture, honey, almond butter, vanilla extract, ground cinnamon, and salt. In order to fully include all of the ingredients, mix well.
3. Shape the mixture into small bite-sized balls, about 1 inch in diameter.
4. Roll each bite in the unsweetened shredded coconut until coated.
5. Place the coated bites on a baking sheet or a plate.
6. Refrigerate the bites for about 30 minutes to firm up.

7. Once they are set, serve and enjoy.

Nutritional Benefits for Seniors:
- Almonds: A source of healthy fats, protein, and essential nutrients that support cognitive and heart health.
- Dried Blueberries: Provide antioxidants and potential cognitive and heart health benefits.
- Honey: Adds natural sweetness and potential anti-inflammatory properties.
- Almond Butter: Contains healthy fats, protein, and essential nutrients for cognitive and heart health.
- Cinnamon: A spice that adds flavor and potential health benefits.
- Coconut: Offers healthy fats and flavor.

These Almond and Blueberry Bites are a delightful and nutritious snack for seniors. They combine the nuttiness of almonds with the sweetness of dried blueberries and a hint of cinnamon. The unsweetened shredded coconut adds a delightful crunch. They make for a wholesome and convenient treat.

Walnut and Banana Muffins

Time of Preparation: 30 minutes

Ingredients:

- 1 1/2 cups all-purpose flour
- 1/2 cup whole wheat flour
- 1 teaspoon baking powder
- 1/2 teaspoon baking soda
- 1/2 teaspoon salt
- 1/2 cup unsalted butter, softened
- 1 cup granulated sugar
- 2 large ripe bananas, mashed
- 2 large eggs
- 1 teaspoon vanilla extract
- 1/2 cup chopped walnuts
- 1/4 cup milk

Method of Preparation:

1. Preheat your oven to 350°F (175°C). Grease the cups or use paper liners to line a muffin pan.
2. In a mixing bowl, combine the all-purpose flour, whole wheat flour, baking powder, baking soda, and salt.
3. In another bowl, cream together the softened unsalted butter and granulated sugar until light and fluffy.
4. Beat in the mashed bananas, eggs, and vanilla extract until well combined.

5. Gradually add the dry ingredients to the banana mixture, alternating with the milk, beginning and ending with the dry ingredients.

6. Fold in the chopped walnuts.

7. Spoon the batter into the prepared muffin cups, filling each about two-thirds full.

8. Bake for about 18 to 20 minutes in a preheated oven, or until a toothpick inserted into the centre of a muffin comes out clean.

9. Remove from the oven and allow the muffins to cool in the tin for a few minutes before transferring them to a wire rack to cool completely.

Nutritional Benefits for Seniors:

- Bananas: A source of vitamins, minerals, and dietary fiber that support cognitive health and digestive function.

- Walnuts: Provide omega-3 fatty acids, antioxidants, and essential nutrients that support cognitive and heart health.

- Whole Wheat Flour: Contains fiber, vitamins, and minerals for digestive health and cognitive function.

These Walnut and Banana Muffins are a delicious and nutritious treat for seniors. They combine the sweetness of ripe bananas with the crunch of chopped walnuts. The use of whole wheat flour adds a bit of wholesome goodness to these muffins. They make for a delightful addition to breakfast or a snack.

Oatmeal Raisin Cookies with Flaxseeds

Time of Preparation: 30 minutes

Ingredients:

- 1 cup old-fashioned oats
- 3/4 cup all-purpose flour
- 1/4 cup ground flaxseeds
- 1/2 teaspoon baking soda
- 1/2 teaspoon ground cinnamon
- 1/4 teaspoon salt
- 1/2 cup unsalted butter, softened
- 1/2 cup brown sugar
- 1/4 cup granulated sugar
- 1 large egg
- 1 teaspoon vanilla extract
- 1/2 cup raisins

Method of Preparation:

1. Preheat your oven to 350°F (175°C). Line a baking sheet with parchment paper.
2. In a mixing bowl, combine the old-fashioned oats, all-purpose flour, ground flaxseeds, baking soda, ground cinnamon, and salt. Mix well.
3. In a separate bowl, cream together the softened unsalted butter, brown sugar, and granulated sugar until the mixture is light and fluffy.

4. Using an egg beater, thoroughly mix in the vanilla essence.

5. Gradually add the dry ingredients to the butter mixture and mix until the dough comes together.

6. Fold in the raisins.

7. Drop spoonfuls of cookie dough onto the prepared baking sheet, leaving some space between each cookie.

8. Flatten each cookie slightly with the back of a spoon or your fingertips.

9. Bake in the preheated oven for approximately 10-12 minutes, or until the cookies are lightly golden.

10. After taking the cookies out of the oven, let them rest for a few minutes on the baking sheet before moving them to a wire rack to finish cooling.

Nutritional Benefits for Seniors:

- Oats: A source of fiber, vitamins, and minerals that support digestive health and cognitive function.

- Flaxseeds: Provide omega-3 fatty acids, fiber, and essential nutrients that support cognitive and heart health.

- Raisins: Offer natural sweetness, vitamins, and antioxidants.

These Oatmeal Raisin Cookies with Flaxseeds are a wholesome and tasty treat for seniors. They combine the nutty flavor of flaxseeds with the sweetness of raisins and the heartiness of oats. They make a delightful and nutritious snack for anytime enjoyment.

Berry and Greek Yogurt Popsicles

Time of Preparation: 10 minutes (including freezing time)

Ingredients:

- 1 cup mixed berries (e.g., strawberries, blueberries, raspberries)
- 1 cup low-fat Greek yogurt
- 2 tablespoons honey (adjust to taste)
- 1/2 teaspoon vanilla extract

Method of Preparation:

1. In a blender, combine the mixed berries, low-fat Greek yogurt, honey, and vanilla extract.
2. Blend until you have a smooth mixture.
3. Taste the mixture and adjust the sweetness with more honey if needed.
4. Pour the mixture into popsicle molds.
5. Insert popsicle sticks into each mold.
6. Freeze for at least 4 hours or until the popsicles are completely frozen.
7. To remove the popsicles from the molds, briefly run them under warm water to loosen.

Nutritional Benefits for Seniors:

- Berries (Strawberries, Blueberries, Raspberries): Rich in vitamins, minerals, and antioxidants that protect brain cells and promote cognitive function.
- Greek Yogurt: A source of protein, probiotics, and calcium, essential for muscle, digestive, and bone health.
- Honey: Adds natural sweetness and potential anti-inflammatory properties.

These Berry and Greek Yogurt Popsicles are a refreshing and nutritious treat for seniors. They combine the goodness of mixed berries with the creaminess of Greek yogurt and a touch of honey. They're perfect for cooling down on a hot day or enjoying as a guilt-free dessert.

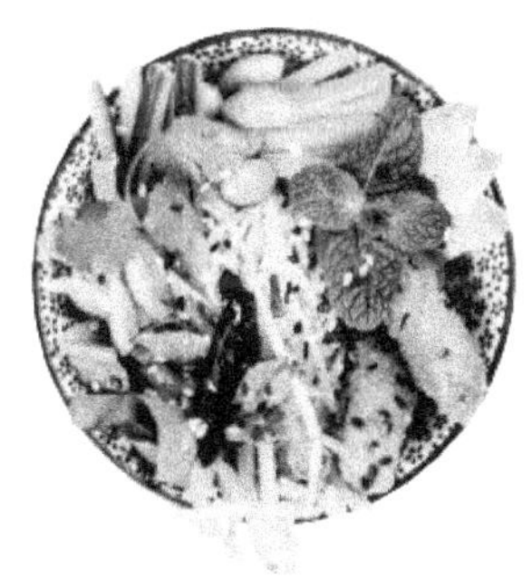

Chapter 8: Beverages

Green Tea with Lemon and Honey

Time of Preparation: 5 minutes

Ingredients:

- 1 green tea bag
- 1 cup hot water
- 1/2 lemon, juiced
- 1-2 teaspoons honey (adjust to taste)

Method of Preparation:

1. Put a bag of green tea into a cup.
2. Pour hot water over the tea bag.
3. Allow the tea to steep for 3-5 minutes, or until it reaches your desired strength.
4. Remove the tea bag.
5. Add freshly squeezed lemon juice to the tea.
6. Stir in honey to sweeten the tea to your liking.
7. Stir until the honey is fully dissolved.
8. Serve the green tea with lemon and honey hot or over ice, depending on your preference.

Nutritional Benefits for Seniors:
- Green Tea: Contains antioxidants and compounds that may support cognitive function and overall health.

- Lemon: A source of vitamin C and antioxidants that promote immune health and protect brain cells.
- Honey: Adds natural sweetness and potential anti-inflammatory properties.

This Green Tea with Lemon and Honey is a soothing and healthy beverage for seniors. It combines the freshness of lemon and the natural sweetness of honey with the antioxidant properties of green tea. It's a comforting choice for a relaxing and revitalizing drink.

Berry and Ginger Infused Water

Time of Preparation: 5 minutes (plus infusing time)

Ingredients:

- 1 cup mixed berries (e.g., strawberries, blueberries, raspberries)
– One thin slice of raw ginger
- 1-2 cups water
- Ice cubes (optional)

Method of Preparation:

1. Rinse the mixed berries and place them in a pitcher.
2. Add the sliced fresh ginger to the berries.
3. Pour water into the pitcher, covering the berries and ginger.

4. Gently muddle the berries and ginger with a muddler or the back of a spoon to release their flavors.
5. Cover the pitcher and refrigerate for at least 2-4 hours or overnight to allow the flavors to infuse.
6. When serving, you can strain the infused water or serve it with the berries and ginger slices for added flavor.
7. Add ice cubes if desired for a refreshing chill.

Nutritional Benefits for Seniors:
- Berries (Strawberries, Blueberries, Raspberries): Rich in vitamins, minerals, and antioxidants that protect brain cells and promote cognitive function.
- Ginger: An herb with potential anti-inflammatory and digestive benefits.

This Berry and Ginger Infused Water is a refreshing and hydrating beverage for seniors. It combines the natural sweetness and antioxidants of mixed berries with the spiciness of fresh ginger. The result is a delightful and healthy way to enjoy your daily water intake.

Turmeric Latte with Cinnamon

Time of Preparation: 10 minutes

Ingredients:

- 1 cup milk of your choice (e.g., dairy milk, almond milk, coconut milk)
- 1/2 teaspoon ground turmeric
- 1/4 teaspoon ground cinnamon
- 1 teaspoon honey (adjust to taste)
- A pinch of ground black pepper (optional)
- A small cinnamon stick for garnish (optional)

Method of Preparation:

1. In a small saucepan, warm the milk over low to medium heat. Be careful not to boil it.
2. Stir in the ground turmeric and ground cinnamon.
3. Add honey to the milk and continue to stir until all the ingredients are well combined.
4. If you like, you can add a pinch of ground black pepper, which may enhance the absorption of curcumin in turmeric.
5. Once the mixture is heated and well-mixed, remove it from the heat.
6. Pour the turmeric latte into a cup.
7. Garnish with a small cinnamon stick if desired.
8. Serve hot.

Nutritional Benefits for Seniors:
- Turmeric: Contains curcumin, which has potential anti-inflammatory and antioxidant properties.
- Cinnamon: An aromatic spice that may help regulate blood sugar levels and provide antioxidant benefits.
- Honey: Adds natural sweetness and potential anti-inflammatory properties.

This Turmeric Latte with Cinnamon is a warming and soothing beverage for seniors. It combines the earthy flavor of turmeric with the warmth of cinnamon and the sweetness of honey. It's a comforting choice for a relaxing and healthy drink.

Herbal Chamomile Tea

Time of Preparation: 5 minutes

Ingredients:

- 1 chamomile tea bag
- 1 cup hot water
- Honey or lemon (optional, for flavor)

Method of Preparation:

1. Place a chamomile tea bag in a cup.
2. Pour hot water over the tea bag.

3. Allow the tea to steep for about 3-5 minutes or until it reaches your desired strength.
4. Remove the tea bag.
5. If you prefer, you can add honey or a squeeze of lemon for extra flavor.
6. Stir to combine if you've added honey.
7. Serve and enjoy your soothing chamomile tea.

Nutritional Benefits for Seniors:
- Chamomile: An herb known for its potential calming and anti-inflammatory properties. It may aid with relaxation and sleep.

Herbal Chamomile Tea is a gentle and relaxing beverage for seniors. Chamomile is well-known for its soothing qualities, making it an excellent choice for winding down and promoting a sense of calm. It's a wonderful way to enjoy a peaceful moment.

Coconut Water and Pineapple Smoothie

Time of Preparation: 5 minutes

Ingredients:

- 1 cup coconut water
- One cup of pineapple pieces, either fresh or frozen
- 1/2 cup Greek yoghurt (to add creaminess, if desired)
- 1 tablespoon honey (adjust to taste)

- Ice cubes (optional)
- Fresh mint leaves for garnish (optional)

Method of Preparation:

1. In a blender, combine the coconut water, pineapple chunks, Greek yogurt (if using), and honey.
2. If you prefer a colder smoothie, you can add ice cubes to the blender as well.
3. Blend until you have a smooth and creamy mixture.
4. After tasting the smoothie, add additional honey if necessary to regulate the sweetness.
5. Transfer smoothie mixture into glass.
6. If preferred, garnish with fresh mint leaves.
7. Serve immediately.

Nutritional Benefits for Seniors:
- Coconut Water: A natural source of hydration, containing electrolytes and essential nutrients.
- Pineapple: Rich in vitamins, minerals, and antioxidants that promote immune health and protect brain cells.
- Greek Yogurt: A source of protein, probiotics, and calcium, essential for muscle, digestive, and bone health.
- Honey: Adds natural sweetness and potential anti-inflammatory properties.

This Coconut Water and Pineapple Smoothie is a refreshing and hydrating choice for seniors. It combines the natural sweetness of pineapple with the tropical essence of coconut water. The addition of Greek yogurt gives it a creamy touch. It's a perfect way to enjoy a nutritious and revitalizing drink.

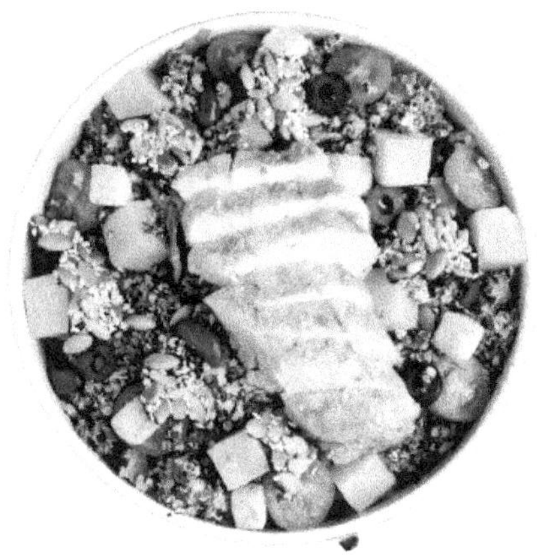

Chapter 9: The Importance of Physical Activity

Physical activity is of paramount importance, especially for seniors, as it offers a wide range of physical and mental health benefits. Here are some key reasons why physical activity is crucial for seniors:

1. Maintaining Physical Health: Regular physical activity helps seniors maintain a healthy weight, strengthen muscles and bones, and improve cardiovascular health. It can reduce the risk of chronic conditions like heart disease, diabetes, and osteoporosis.

2. Enhancing Mobility and Balance: Physical activity, including exercises like walking, yoga, and tai chi, can improve balance, flexibility, and mobility. This is essential for preventing falls and maintaining independence.

3. Cognitive Function: Studies suggest that physical activity may support cognitive function and reduce the risk of cognitive decline and dementia. It can enhance memory, problem-solving skills, and overall mental sharpness.

4. Mood and Mental Health: Exercise releases endorphins, which can elevate mood and reduce the risk of depression and anxiety. It offers a natural way to cope with stress and boost mental well-being.

5. Social Interaction: Many forms of physical activity, such as group classes or team sports, provide opportunities for social interaction. Maintaining social connections is crucial for mental health, particularly in later years.

6. Better Sleep: Regular physical activity can help seniors improve the quality of their sleep. It can reduce insomnia and promote restful, restorative sleep.

7. Chronic Disease Management: For seniors living with chronic conditions, physical activity can be an integral part of managing their health. It can help control symptoms and improve overall well-being.

8. Independence: By maintaining physical fitness and mobility, seniors can continue to perform daily activities independently. This self-sufficiency is essential for their quality of life.

9. Pain Management: Exercise can help reduce chronic pain associated with conditions like arthritis and back problems. It strengthens the body and provides better support for joints.

10. Longevity: Engaging in regular physical activity has been linked to a longer and healthier life. It can delay the onset of age-related health issues and improve overall life expectancy.

It's important for seniors to choose physical activities that suit their abilities and interests. Consulting with a healthcare provider or a fitness expert can help create a tailored exercise plan. Regardless of the chosen activities, incorporating regular movement and exercise into daily life is one of the best ways for seniors to maintain their health and well-being.

Stress Reduction and Memory improvement

Stress reduction and memory improvement are interconnected and essential aspects of maintaining cognitive health and overall well-being, especially for seniors. Here's how managing stress can lead to memory enhancement:

Stress Reduction and Memory Improvement:

1. Cortisol Regulation: Chronic stress can lead to elevated levels of the stress hormone cortisol, which can impair memory and cognitive function. By managing stress, you can help regulate cortisol levels, leading to improved memory.

2. Enhanced Concentration: Stress often leads to distraction and difficulty in focusing. Reducing stress through relaxation techniques like meditation or mindfulness can enhance your ability to concentrate, which is crucial for memory retention.

3. Better Sleep: Stress can disrupt sleep patterns and affect the consolidation of memories during deep sleep. Stress reduction strategies, such as relaxation exercises, can improve the quality of your sleep, facilitating better memory retention.

4. Brain Health: Chronic stress may contribute to the shrinking of the hippocampus, a brain region critical for memory formation. Managing stress can help preserve the integrity of this brain structure.

5. Mood Improvement: Stress often accompanies negative moods and emotions, which can affect memory negatively. Reducing stress can lead to a more positive outlook and improved memory recall.

Effective Stress Reduction Techniques for Memory Improvement:

1. Meditation and Mindfulness: These practices can help calm the mind, reduce stress, and improve memory by enhancing focus and cognitive function.

2. Regular Exercise: Physical activity has been linked to stress reduction and cognitive improvement. It promotes the release of endorphins, which elevate mood and reduce stress.

3. Adequate Sleep: Prioritizing sleep and maintaining a regular sleep schedule is vital for managing stress and enhancing memory.

4. Balanced Diet: Nutrient-rich foods, particularly those high in antioxidants and omega-3 fatty acids, can support brain health and reduce the impact of stress.

5. Social Interaction: Spending time with friends and family and participating in social activities can help alleviate stress and stimulate cognitive functions.

6. Relaxation Techniques: Deep breathing exercises, progressive muscle relaxation, and other relaxation techniques can help manage stress effectively.

7. Cognitive Training: Engaging in mentally stimulating activities like puzzles, games, or learning new skills can improve memory and reduce stress.

8. Professional Support: If stress is overwhelming, it's essential to seek the support of a mental health professional who can provide counseling or therapy.

It's important for seniors to adopt a holistic approach to managing stress and improving memory. Lifestyle changes, relaxation techniques, and a supportive social network can all contribute to reducing stress and enhancing cognitive function, leading to a better quality of life in the later years.

Social Engagement and Brain Health

Social engagement plays a crucial role in maintaining brain health, especially for seniors. It offers a wide range of cognitive, emotional, and physical benefits that can contribute to a higher quality of life in later years. Here's how social engagement positively affects brain health:

1. Cognitive Stimulation: Engaging in conversations, participating in group activities, and interacting with others provide continuous cognitive stimulation. These interactions challenge the brain and help keep it active and agile.

2. Mood Improvement: Socializing and forming connections with friends and family members often lead to improved mood and reduced feelings of loneliness and depression. A positive mood is linked to better cognitive function.

3. Stress Reduction: Meaningful social connections can act as a buffer against stress. Reducing stress is essential for maintaining cognitive health.

4. Intellectual Growth: Social activities often involve learning, problem-solving, and decision-making. This intellectual growth can contribute to enhanced cognitive function and memory.

5. Enhanced Memory: Engaging in conversations and storytelling with others can improve memory recall and verbal skills.

6. Emotional Support: Having a support system in the form of social connections can provide emotional security and resilience. This emotional well-being is connected to cognitive health.

7. Physical Health: Social engagement often involves physical activity, such as walking, dancing, or group exercise classes. Regular physical activity supports brain health.

8. Chronic Disease Management: Social interactions can provide encouragement and support for seniors managing chronic conditions, leading to better overall well-being.

Ways to Promote Social Engagement

1. Join Clubs or Groups: Participate in clubs, organizations, or groups related to personal interests, hobbies, or volunteering opportunities.

2. Stay Connected: Maintain contact with friends and family through phone calls, video chats, or in-person visits.

3. Attend Senior Centers: Senior centers often offer a variety of activities and social programs to connect with peers.

4. Community Involvement: Get involved in community events, local classes, or cultural activities.

5. Support Networks: Seek support groups for specific health conditions or personal interests.

6. Technology Use: Embrace technology to connect with others through social media or online communities.

7. Hobbies and Interests: Pursue hobbies and interests that encourage interaction with others, such as book clubs or art classes.

8. Family Gatherings: Organize and attend family gatherings and celebrations to foster meaningful connections.

Maintaining social engagement is an integral part of a healthy and fulfilling life for seniors. It contributes to cognitive vitality, emotional well-being, and physical health. Seniors are encouraged to explore various avenues for social interaction and build meaningful connections with others to promote brain health and overall quality of life.

Supporting Loved ones with Memory Loss

Supporting loved ones with memory loss, particularly for seniors, is a significant responsibility that requires empathy, patience, and understanding. Here are a few helpful methods for giving support:

1. Educate Yourself: Learn about the specific memory condition your loved one is dealing with, whether it's dementia, Alzheimer's disease, or another form of memory loss. Having knowledge of the problem will enable you to offer suitable assistance.

2. Effective Communication: Use clear, simple, and direct communication. Talk gently and deliberately while maintaining eye contact. Allow your loved one time to process and respond to conversations.

3. Maintain Routine: Establish and maintain a consistent daily routine. Predictable schedules can reduce confusion and anxiety.

4. Memory Aids: Use memory aids like calendars, notes, and reminders to help your loved one keep track of important dates and tasks.

5. Be Patient: Be patient and understanding when your loved one repeats themselves or forgets things. Avoid correcting or arguing with them.

6. Encourage Independence: Promote independence by allowing your loved one to do as much as they can for themselves. Provide support when needed but avoid doing everything for them.

7. Safe Environment: Ensure the home environment is safe by removing tripping hazards and making necessary modifications to accommodate their needs.

8. Nutritious Diet: Offer a well-balanced diet that supports brain health. Omega-3 fatty acids, antioxidants, and nutrient-dense foods can be beneficial.

9. Regular Exercise: Encourage regular physical activity, as it can help maintain physical and cognitive function. Activities like walking or gentle yoga are often suitable.

10. Social Interaction: Promote social engagement to combat loneliness and depression. Encourage participation in social activities, family gatherings, and support groups.

11. Memory Exercises: Engage your loved one in memory exercises and brain-stimulating activities, such as puzzles, games, and reading.

12. Seek Professional Help: Consult with healthcare professionals for diagnosis, treatment, and guidance. Medications and therapies may be recommended.

13. Respite Care: Consider respite care to provide you with a break while ensuring your loved one receives the necessary care.

14. Self-Care: Caring for someone with memory loss can be emotionally and physically draining. Make sure to prioritize your own well-being and seek support for yourself, too.

15. Legal and Financial Planning: Ensure legal and financial matters are in order, including wills, powers of attorney, and financial planning. Seek legal advice if necessary.

16. Quality Time: Spend quality time together doing activities your loved one enjoys. Create positive memories and experiences.

17. Empathy and Compassion: Approach caregiving with empathy and compassion. Understand that your loved one may feel frustration, fear, or sadness due to memory loss.

18. Support Network: Build a support network with family, friends, or support groups. It's essential to share the responsibilities and seek advice from others who have experienced similar situations.

Supporting a loved one with memory loss can be challenging, but it's also an opportunity to provide care, comfort, and love. Remember that you're making a positive difference in their life by being there for them and ensuring they have the best possible quality of life despite their memory condition.

Meal Preparation Strategies for Caregivers

Meal preparation for caregivers is essential, especially when caring for loved ones with memory loss or other health issues. Here are some meal preparation strategies to make this task more manageable:

1. Meal Planning:

- Plan meals in advance to ensure a balanced and nutritious diet.
- Create a weekly menu that includes a variety of foods from different food groups.
- Take into account any dietary restrictions or preferences your loved one may have.

2. Simplify Recipes:

- Choose simple, easy-to-follow recipes that don't require complex cooking techniques.
- Opt for one-pot meals or slow cooker recipes that minimize the number of dishes and steps involved.

3. Prep Ingredients in Advance:

- Wash, chop, and prepare ingredients ahead of time to save time during meal preparation.
- Store prepped ingredients in labeled containers to make cooking easier.

4. Freeze Meals:

- Cook larger batches of meals and freeze individual portions for future use. This is especially helpful for days when you may not have time to cook.

5. Use Convenience Foods:
- Utilize healthy convenience foods like pre-cut vegetables, canned beans, or frozen fruits and vegetables.
- These can reduce prep time while still providing nutritional value.

6. Label and Date Food:
- Label containers with the date of preparation to ensure freshness.
- This is important, especially if you prepare meals in advance.

7. Portion Control:
- Consider using portion control containers to manage portion sizes, especially if your loved one needs specific dietary restrictions.

8. Hydration:
- Ensure your loved one stays hydrated by having water and other preferred beverages readily available.

9. Include Snacks:
- Prepare healthy and easy-to-access snacks, such as fruit slices, yogurt, or nuts, for between meals.

10. Dietary Considerations:

- Be aware of any dietary restrictions or needs your loved one has, such as allergies, diabetes, or heart health concerns.
- Seek advice from a nutritionist or medical professional.

11. Safety First:

- If your loved one has memory issues, ensure that the kitchen is safe by removing potential hazards and supervising when necessary.

12. Serve Familiar Foods:

- Stick to familiar and favorite foods to make mealtime more enjoyable and reduce resistance to new dishes.

13. Scheduled Meals:

- Establish regular mealtime schedules to create a routine that your loved one can rely on.

14. Encourage Independence:

- If possible, involve your loved one in meal preparation to maintain a sense of independence. They can assist with simple tasks.

15. Monitor Changes:

- Keep an eye on any changes in appetite, preferences, or dietary needs and adjust meal planning accordingly.

16. Seek Support:

- Don't hesitate to ask for help from other family members or consider professional caregiving services to share the responsibilities.

17. Self-Care:

-Do not overlook the need of self-care. Caregiving can be demanding, and you need to maintain your well-being to provide the best care.

Remember that meal preparation for caregivers is not just about providing nutrition but also about creating a positive and comfortable dining experience for your loved one. Tailoring your approach to their specific needs and preferences is essential for their overall well-being.

Conclusion

In conclusion, "The Memory Loss Recuperation Cookbook for Seniors for Seniors" is more than just a collection of recipes; it's a heartfelt journey into the world of nurturing the mind and body. It has been our pleasure to embark on this culinary exploration, guided by the belief that the power of nutrition and connection is a path to not only managing memory loss but also savoring life's moments.

Through these pages, we've discovered the importance of understanding memory loss and the significance of nutrition for brain health. We've explored 40 brain-enhancing recipes that are not only delicious but also packed with nutrients to support cognitive function.

We've delved into the art of meal preparation for caregivers, recognizing that caregivers play a pivotal role in the well-being of their loved ones. We've explored strategies to enhance emotional well-being for caregivers, acknowledging that self-care and support networks are essential on this journey.

We've celebrated the role of social engagement and the positive impact it has on brain health. The stories shared and the strategies presented here remind us that we are never alone on this path. Our interconnectedness and the power of the human spirit provide the strength to face the challenges of memory loss.

In the end, "The Memory Loss Recuperation Cookbook for Seniors" is a testament to the human spirit's resilience, the nourishment of body and soul, and the beauty of savoring every moment. It is our hope that this book serves as a source of guidance, inspiration, and delicious meals that contribute to a brighter, healthier, and more meaningful journey for seniors and their caregivers.

May this cookbook be a tool for creating not only nutritious and delightful dishes but also lasting memories, and may it illuminate the path toward a life well-lived, regardless of the challenges of memory loss.

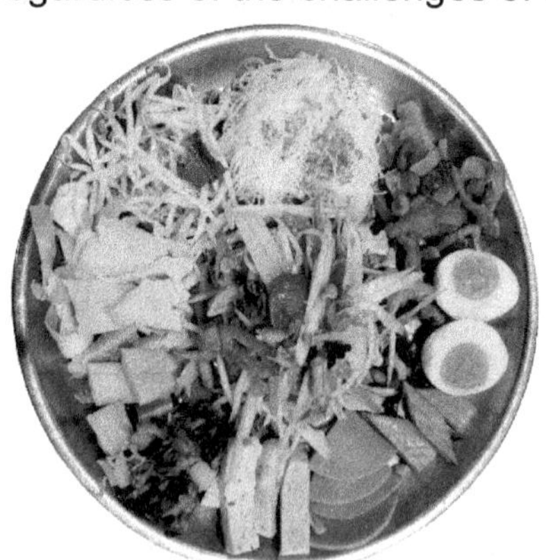